W0227577

The Welfare Workforce

The Welfare Workforce is a thought-provoking exploration of mental health care in the United States and beyond. Although all the affluent democracies pursued deinstitutionalization, some failed to provide adequate services, while others overcame challenges of stigma and limited resources and successfully expanded care. Isabel M. Perera examines the role of the "welfare workforce" in providing social services to those who cannot demand them. Drawing on extensive research in four countries – the United States, France, Norway, and Sweden – Perera sheds light on postindustrial politics and the critical part played by those who work for the welfare state. A must-read for anyone interested in mental health care, social services, and the politics of welfare, *The Welfare Workforce* challenges conventional wisdom and offers new insights into the complex factors that contribute to the success or failure of mental health care systems. This title is also available as Open Access on Cambridge Core.

Isabel M. Perera is an assistant professor in the Department of Government at Cornell University. Perera has held visiting positions at the European University Institute, the University of Gothenburg, the University of Oxford, and Sciences Po Paris. This book is based on her award-winning dissertation in political science written at the University of Pennsylvania. Her academic training also includes a postdoctoral fellowship in health policy and medical ethics.

Cambridge Studies in Comparative Politics

General Editor

Kathleen Thelen, *Massachusetts Institute of Technology*

Associate Editors

Lisa Blaydes, *Stanford University*
Catherine Boone, *London School of Economics and Political Science*
Thad Dunning, *University of California, Berkeley*
Anna Grzymala-Busse, *Stanford University*
Torben Iversen, *Harvard University*
Stathis Kalyvas, *University of Oxford*
Melanie Manion, *Duke University*
Prerna Singh, *Brown University*
Dan Slater, *University of Michigan*
Susan Stokes, *Yale University*
Tariq Thachil, *University of Pennsylvania*
Erik Wibbels, *University of Pennsylvania*

Series Founder

Peter Lange, *Duke University*

Editor Emeritus

Margaret Levi, *Stanford University*

Other Books in the Series

Christopher Adolph, *Bankers, Bureaucrats, and Central Bank Politics: The Myth of Neutrality*
Michael Albertus, *Autocracy and Redistribution: The Politics of Land Reform*
Michael Albertus, *Property without Rights: Origins and Consequences of the Property Rights Gap*
Santiago Anria, *When Movements Become Parties: The Bolivian MAS in Comparative Perspective*
Ben W. Ansell, *From the Ballot to the Blackboard: The Redistributive Political Economy of Education*
Ben W. Ansell and Johannes Lindvall, *Inward Conquest: The Political Origins of Modern Public Services*
Ben W. Ansell and David J. Samuels, *Inequality and Democratization: An Elite-Competition Approach*
Ana Arjona, *Rebelocracy: Social Order in the Colombian Civil War*
Leonardo R. Arriola, *Multi-Ethnic Coalitions in Africa: Business Financing of Opposition Election Campaigns*

(continued after index)

The Welfare Workforce

Why Mental Health Care Varies Across Affluent Democracies

ISABEL M. PERERA

Cornell University

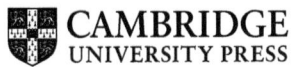

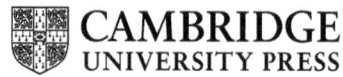

Shaftesbury Road, Cambridge CB2 8EA, United Kingdom

One Liberty Plaza, 20th Floor, New York, NY 10006, USA

477 Williamstown Road, Port Melbourne, VIC 3207, Australia

314–321, 3rd Floor, Plot 3, Splendor Forum, Jasola District Centre, New Delhi – 110025, India

103 Penang Road, #05–06/07, Visioncrest Commercial, Singapore 238467

Cambridge University Press is part of Cambridge University Press & Assessment, a department of the University of Cambridge.

We share the University's mission to contribute to society through the pursuit of education, learning and research at the highest international levels of excellence.

www.cambridge.org
Information on this title: www.cambridge.org/9781009499897

DOI: 10.1017/9781009499866

© Isabel M. Perera 2025

This publication is in copyright. Subject to statutory exception and to the provisions of relevant collective licensing agreements, with the exception of the Creative Commons version the link for which is provided below, no reproduction of any part may take place without the written permission of Cambridge University Press & Assessment.

An online version of this work is published at doi.org/10.1017/9781009499866 under a Creative Commons Open Access license CC-BY-NC 4.0 which permits re-use, distribution and reproduction in any medium for non-commercial purposes providing appropriate credit to the original work is given and any changes made are indicated. To view a copy of this license visit https://creativecommons.org/licenses/by-nc/4.0

When citing this work, please include a reference to the DOI 10.1017/9781009499866

First published 2025

A catalogue record for this publication is available from the British Library

A Cataloging-in-Publication data record for this book is available from the Library of Congress

ISBN 978-1-009-49989-7 Hardback
ISBN 978-1-009-49984-2 Paperback

Cambridge University Press & Assessment has no responsibility for the persistence or accuracy of URLs for external or third-party internet websites referred to in this publication and does not guarantee that any content on such websites is, or will remain, accurate or appropriate.

Contents

Figures

Tables

Preface

This book began with a midnight shriek. It was loud, piercing, and desperate, the kind that makes you realize that something has gone irreparably wrong. The sound had reached my window, high on the tenth floor of an apartment building in downtown Philadelphia. As the howling continued, I inched closer to the window to discern its origins. There was a man circling the street corner, with movements that seemed to fluctuate between fury and fantasy. He was experiencing, it seemed, a psychotic episode.

While his mind paced, so did mine. Where could he go? Although this "public disturbance" might warrant a police arrest, surely that was not the most appropriate response. His needs seemed medical. A nearby health clinic? I didn't know of any that could provide the level of psychiatric attention he required; and besides, most were closed by now. The emergency room? A single overnight stay might not be sufficient. I wondered, too, where he lived, whether he was able to keep a job, and to what extent his family could support him. The answers to these questions, I imagined, would likely disappoint. Comprehensive and long-term care for people with severe psychiatric conditions is difficult and expensive to obtain in the United States.

As a scholar of the comparative politics of social policy, I began to investigate mental health systems, both in the United States and in other countries. What might this man's options have been in Paris, Stockholm, or Oslo? The answer was surprising. Psychiatric deinstitutionalization, whose mishandling US observers often blamed for their system's contemporary ills, had occurred in parallel across the affluent democracies. All of them had transformed mental health care systems by depopulating residential psychiatric hospitals. Similar social movements, pharmaceutical developments, and fiscal changes had pressured these countries to reduce hospital-based care. But the results of these reforms varied widely. In some countries, such as the United States, policy-makers closed hospitals but failed to replace them with adequate social and medical supports. Other countries, though, developed much more expansive public mental health care systems. Moreover, contemporary mental health care seemed unrelated to general health care, as in the example of France, which developed public sector psychiatry despite the country's long tradition of private general practice. It also seemed unrelated to other forms of social service provision. For example, although Norway and Sweden both tend to provide extensive, Scandinavian-style public services in most policy areas, the supply of public mental health care is much higher in Norway than in Sweden. From a political and economic standpoint, the high supply of services in some countries was puzzling because their beneficiaries rarely requested them; people with chronic and severe mental illness are the subjects of significant political, social, and economic disenfranchisement. Thus I arrived at the central empirical and theoretical questions that drive this book project: What explains the cross-national variation in mental health care services? And why, then, would the state supply services to those who are unable to demand them?

A potential answer appeared as I combed through the French archives. The Syndicat des médecins des hôpitaux psychiatriques (Trade Union of Psychiatric Hospital Physicians) seemed pivotal to every important mental health policy decision since the onset of deinstitutionalization. This group was unlike other associations of physicians. It was a trade union; and its members spent much of their time managing public institutions. Protecting government-funded psychiatric services – and their employees – was central to the trade union's mission. Nurses, attendants, and social workers, also represented by trade unions, were close coalition partners. Although patient advocacy was limited, the coalition between organized managers and workers in the public sector served as a political counterweight to the financial pressure to reduce services, advancing policies that both protected their employment and broadened the spectrum of care. Yes, France deinstitutionalized the mentally ill in the late 20th century; but it did so by expanding outpatient services, not by closing most of its hospitals.

The timing of these events, I soon realized, was no coincidence. Mental health workers gained political influence precisely as other service sector employees gained a greater share of overall employment. In 1960, the average western democracy employed about the same share of workers in industry and in services (about 37 and 41 percent, respectively). Today, service sector employment has nearly doubled (to 78 percent), while industrial employment has halved (to 20 percent) (Brady et al. 2020, author's calculations). Employment in social services, in particular, underpinned much of this transition, as countries began to expand their health, education, and social care systems. The effects were both personal and political, and sometimes experienced over a single generation. If the postwar worker had found employment in an auto plant, his daughter might find it in a hospital. Moreover, if his representative trade unions once sought to protect the car industry, hers now seek to expand the health sector. Such were the claims that arose across the affluent democracies during deinstitutionalization. By the late 20th century, the growing numbers of workers employed by the welfare state – what I call the "welfare workforce" – had become a significant actor in its politics.

Viewed against this backdrop, the transformation of mental health care is a window into how government employees are shaping social policy. This book examines both these subjects. Empirically, I document the historical and contemporary variations in mental health care services across the affluent democracies, tracing how coalitions of public sector managers and workers drove the expansion of services in France and Norway, while their absence in the United States and Sweden produced the opposite outcomes in those countries. Theoretically, I explore a new distributive logic of welfare provision. In striking contrast to the postwar period, it is public sector, not private sector, unions that now often shape social policy. I investigate when, why, and how they gain influence, and with what implications for those the welfare state promises to serve.

Acknowledgments

Since that fateful evening in Philadelphia, this project has benefited from over a decade of guidance, feedback, and assistance from others. Thanks go first to Julia Lynch, my doctoral advisor at Penn, whose exacting standards and singular energy pushed the research to new heights. Well-timed conversations with my formal committee members, Dawn Teele and Marie Gottschalk, as well as my acting supervisors while abroad, Jane Gingrich and Desmond King, also played significant roles at pivotal moments in graduate school. A postdoctoral fellowship with Dominic Sisti at Penn's medical school then opened doors to audiences and opportunities beyond my expectations.

Nor did I expect that the scholars I had read and admired as a student would eventually become my faculty colleagues. But that is what happened when I joined Cornell. Suzanne Mettler has provided outstanding mentorship at every step of the publication process. Sidney Tarrow reviewed the entire manuscript with characteristic generosity and insight. Feedback from Peter Katzenstein on Chapter 1, Richard Bensel and Nicolas van de Walle on Chapter 3, Jamila Michener on Chapter 7, and Gustavo Flores-Macías and Tom Pepinsky on the proposal were targeted interventions with a very big impact. Thanks also go to Rachel Reidl, who sought out a wonderful writing space for me; and to Jill Frank, Jason Frank, and Ken Roberts, the department chairs who ensured a productive research environment.

Essential to this book's completion were several other institutional homes and intellectual communities. Special thanks go to Henri Bergeron for securing the sponsorship of Sciences Po Paris (twice) and to Johannes Lindvall for that of the University of Gothenburg. I also benefited from extended visits to the University of Oxford, the European University Institute, and the Brocher Foundation. Along the way, many additional scholars propelled the project to its final form. In particular, Chapter 5 gained from a helpful discussion with Matthias Brunn, Elisa Chelle, Lucie Kraepiel, Takuya Onoda, and Tonya Tartour, and from comments from Anton Hemerijck; and it remains indebted to Alex Barnard, my fortuitous fieldwork partner. Chapter 6 emerged from the advice of Andrea Campbell and Peter Swenson and materialized with the guidance of Karen Anderson, Frida Boräng, Carl Dahlström, and Jon Pierre.

My academic preoccupation with the costs of labor-intensive work is partially the product of a lived reality. Time, travel, and other assistance for this research was funded by: Cornell University (the Department of Government, the Institute for European Studies, the Qualitative and Interpretive Research Institute, the Humanities Council, and the Toward an Open Monograph Ecosystem [TOME] Initiative); the University of Pennsylvania (the Fontaine, GAPSA-Provost, School of Arts and Sciences Dissertation Research, Mellon Graduate Education, Queen Elizabeth, and Fox Leadership International Alumni Research and Service [FLIARS] fellowships, the Browne and Lauder Centers, and the Department of Medical Ethics and Health Policy); the European University Institute Max Weber Fellowship Program; the Embassy of France in the United States Chateaubriand Program; the Sciences Po Laboratory for Interdisciplinary Evaluation of Public Policies (LIEPP) International Scholars in Policy Evaluation Program; the Société des professeurs français et francophones d'Amérique; the Brocher Foundation Residency Program; and the Horowitz Foundation for Social Policy. These resources made it possible for Josette Barrans, Trevor Brown, Daniel Carelli, Catherine Hendicott, Frida Jonsson, Alyson Price, Samantha Surdek, Aiysha Varraich, and especially, Pia Kohler to contribute their research and editorial assistance as well.

Countless others devoted their valuable time to this project, too. Interviewees and area specialists shared their knowledge and resources; François Chapireau even procured obscure administrative documents when no one else could and then offered feedback on the manuscript. Archivists and librarians provided skilled source assistance; in fact, Stefanie Caloia cannot be thanked enough for making the unprocessed AFSCME collections available to me. Administrators at multiple institutions helped to execute this complex international project; for which Dinnie Sloman and Laurie Dorsey at Cornell graciously bore the brunt of the logistics. Many good friends accompanied me on this long road;

so much so that Danielle Hanley, Tanguy Hubert, and André Victor Doherty Luduvice found themselves providing direct technical and project management support at various points.

Finally, the confidence of my family carried this book from inception to completion. My grandmothers, Bohemia Perera and Mary Solernou, who just missed its publication, know that I often thought of my late grandfathers, Dr. Faustino Perera, Sr. and Dr. Emilio Solernou, Sr., while researching this topic. Their faith in me – and (crucially) that of my uncle, Emilio Solernou, Jr. – never faltered. Above all, I thank my parents, Mariloly Solernou and Tino Perera, the two public sector employees who have influenced me the most.

NOTE ON BOOK

Publication of this open monograph was the result of Cornell University's participation in TOME, a collaboration of the Association of American Universities, the Association of University Presses, and the Association of Research Libraries. TOME aims to expand the reach of long-form humanities and social science scholarship, including digital scholarship. Additionally, the program looks to ensure the sustainability of university press monograph publishing by supporting the highest quality scholarship and promoting a new ecology of scholarly publishing in which authors' institutions bear the publication costs.

Funding from Cornell University made it possible to open this publication to the world.

www.openmonograph.org

Nothing herein set forth shall serve in any way to alter the original Agreement except as specified above. To the extent any terms or conditions of the Agreement conflict with or are inconsistent with this Amendment, the terms of this Amendment will prevail. In agreeing to the terms of this Amendment, both parties accept the terms of the Creative Commons license assigned to the work, as set forth on the Creative Commons website (https://creativecommons.org/licenses/).

Abbreviations

AFL-CIO	American Federation of Labor and Congress of Industrial Organizations
AFSCME	American Federation of State, County, and Municipal Employees
AMA	American Medical Association
APA	American Psychiatric Association
CES	*Certificat d'études supérieures* (Certificate of graduate study)
CFDT	Confédération française démocratique du travail (French Democratic Confederation of Labor)
CGT	Confédération générale du travail (General Confederation of Labor)
CHS	*Centre hospitalier spécialisé* (Specialty hospital)
CHU	*Centre hospitalier universitaire* (Academic hospital)
CMHC	community mental health center
CSMF	Confédération des syndicats médicaux français (Confederation of French Medical Trade Unions)
DDASS	Direction départementale des affaires sanitaires et sociales (*Département*-level agency for health and social affairs)
FO	Force ouvrière (Workers' Force)
GDP	gross domestic product
IMD	institutions for mental disease
IMD Exclusion	Medicaid provision that prohibits payment to IMDs
ISP	*Infirmier de secteur psychiatrique* (Psychiatric sector nurse)

KS	Kommunenes Sentralforbund (Norwegian Association of Local and Regional Authorities)
LSS	*Lag om stöd och service till vissa funktionshindrade* (Law on support and services for certain disabled persons)
NOK	Norwegian krone
NOU	*Norsk offentlig utredning* (Norwegian government official report)
OECD	Organisation for Economic Co-operation and Development
SEK	Swedish krona
SKTF	Sveriges kommunaltjänstemannaförbund (Swedish Municipal Employees Union)
SOU	*Statlig offentlig utredning* (Swedish government official report)
SS(D)I	Social Security (Disability) Insurance
Syndicat	Syndicat des médecins des hôpitaux psychiatriques (Trade Union of Psychiatric Hospital Physicians)
USD	United States dollar
WHO	World Health Organization
YAVIS	young, attractive, verbal, intelligent, and successful (per Schofield 1964)

The Welfare Workforce

Managers and Workers Make Strange Bedfellows

December 28, 2020, was "Demolition Day" at Allentown State Hospital. Nearly ten months into the Covid-19 pandemic, the decision to raze a health care facility might appear counterintuitive. After all, the calls to protect and extend the medical supply had sounded loud and clear. Such calls were especially relevant to a psychiatric service such as this one, where patients faced a high risk of Covid transmission within the hospital but even worse outcomes if discharged. Increasing capacity in order to maintain social distancing among patients was crucial. But in effect the demolition of Allentown State Hospital was the last of a long line of policy changes in mental health care. The facility had been nonoperational for over a decade, following similar closures at the nearby Mayview State Hospital in 2008, the Harrisburg State Hospital in 2006, and a hundred other state mental hospitals across America (SAMHSA 2011; Witkin et al. 1996). Like many of its peers, Allentown State Hospital was over 100 years old and eligible for inclusion in the US National Register of Historic Places. Simply maintaining its 217-acre campus, though, cost the state about $2 million (USD) each year. The hospital's fate, in the end, was lamentable but cost-effective, and not unlike that of most other American public mental health care facilities.

Meanwhile, across the Atlantic, another mental hospital was faring very differently in the pandemic. Just a few months later, in March 2021, the new director of the Centre de Postcure et de Réadaptation de Billiers announced the launch of three new projects: an in-home care service, an expanded vocational training program, and a short-term housing unit to accommodate the expanded clientele. This was on top of the facility's existing services. Located in a small French village on Brittany's western coast, the campus already housed 145 beds, an arts center, and sheltered employment workshops in four areas: agriculture, horticulture, technical fields such as carpentry and mechanics, and dining and hospitality (the site's restaurant and guest accommodation serve as the training ground). The facility also provides each patient with individualized attention from a large team of professionals, including a psychiatrist, a nurse, a psychologist, a neuropsychologist, an occupational therapist, several social workers, several special needs teachers, and even a sports coach. Many of these services are required by law, as this area is home to one of France's approximately 1,200 psychiatric "sectors," which stipulate at least one such care team for about every 60,000–70,000 people (Chevreul et al. 2015; Coldefy et al. 2009).[1] Evidently, mental health care in France did not face the same fate as that of its American counterpart.

Despite the two countries' dissimilar political reputations when it comes to social policy, the explanation for these alternative fates is not obvious. During the pandemic, the US government expanded some social policies, while the French government sought ways to support markets and the private sector. Historically, too, the general health system in France has been similar to that of the United States, insofar as they share a strong tradition of private practice and payment. Moreover, the demand for mental health care is not higher in Billiers than in Allentown. In fact, the opposite may be the case: The population of Allentown is well over 100 times that of the Billiers. If the prevalence of schizophrenia is around half a percent (estimates vary, WHO 2022), Allentown would have over 500 residents in need of long-term psychiatric attention, but Billiers would have just five. Nor is Billiers, and its surrounding region, more financially capable of supplying mental health care. As is so often the case with these services, their high costs are absorbed by the government, where tightening budgets are becoming less likely to accommodate them. Only a few years earlier in 2015, the Breton health authorities had sought to redress an annual structural deficit of €300,000 (about $360,000) by halving care.[2]

There is another important similarity between Allentown State Hospital and the Centre de Postcure: their respective roles as employers

---

[1] For more information on the specific status and role of the Centre de Postcure in the local psychiatric sector (as an "*ESPIC rattaché au secteur*"), see Bénard et al. (2020); de Cadeville (2016).

[2] Throughout the text, I have standardized monetary amounts to US dollars, using exchange rates for contemporary amounts (here, ECB 2022) and, to approximate historic amounts, local price indices and purchasing power parities.

in deindustrializing local economies. The Billy Joel anthem – "Well we're living here in Allentown / And they're closing all the factories down" – might as well apply to Billiers (Joel 1982). Situated between the ports of Saint-Nazaire and Lorient, Billiers can no longer depend on the ship-building, cargo, and naval industries for employment the way it once did; just as Allentown can no longer depend on the coal, steel, textile, and cement industries of the past. In both places, the one-time reliance on industrial production has shifted dramatically to services, especially social services. Jobs at the local psychiatric hospital are some of the few well-paid and protected jobs still left in town.

The difference, as I will demonstrate in this book, lies in the political response of hospital employees to the respective cuts. Even though, prior to its closing, Allentown State Hospital employed more than triple the staff of the Centre de Postcure (379 full-time employees compared to 110), resistance was more limited in Allentown. To be sure, the closure upset the Allentown employees. The state had transferred a quarter of the staff to another facility and left the rest looking for work or otherwise forced to retire. Unions representing the workers, such as the American Federation of State, County, and Municipal Employees and the Service Employees International Union, argued that the state had made this deci-sion without their consent, failing to account for both their members' livelihoods and the fate of the patients who would be sent elsewhere.

Picket signs in Billiers – "Health and Jobs in Danger" – raised similar concerns at the prospect of budget cuts in 2015, but with the opposite result. The Confédération française démocratique du travail, France's largest labor union for public employees, organized a sweeping mobi-lization; 5,000 people signed a petition opposing the cuts. With their supporters, hospital staff marched four kilometers from the Centre de Postcure to the neighboring town of Muzillac and then on to the prefec-ture in Vannes. Alongside them were 17 local mayors. Elected officials had voted unanimously to support the mobilization, even closing a town hall and post office on the same day as an endorsement. The group of workers, unlike their counterparts in the United States, achieved their objectives. "This new future will help to preserve jobs," the local press concluded, "a major advantage of these projects."[3]

---

[3] "Allentown State Hospital: Former Employees Reflect on Its History," *69News WFMZ-TV*, February 25 and 26, 2019; Andrew Wagaman, "The Allentown State Hospital Site Will Be Redeveloped: A New Report Examines Three Buildout Scenarios," *The Morning Call*, March 11, 2021; Bevin Theodore, "Union Members Scheduled to Protest Closing of Allentown State Hospital at Hearing," *The Express-Times*

The contrasting trajectories of mental health care in Billiers and Allentown help to answer a puzzling question of political economy: Why would the government provide social services to clients who cannot demand them? Welfare states have minimal incentives to do so.[4] Not only are the costs of supplying such services extraordinarily high, their beneficiaries rarely request them. Marginalized groups, such as people with chronic and severe mental illness, possess neither the political clout nor the purchasing power to command robust government attention. Other examples abound. Consider the paradoxical, though varied, choice to supply care homes to the frail elderly, health services to noncitizen immigrants, and even schools to nonvoting-age children. In each of these cases, disenfranchised clients cannot compel the welfare state to deliver these expensive services, but it does, sometimes.

The cross-national variation in mental health care, the empirical subject of this book, throws that puzzling theoretical question into stark, pragmatic relief. What occurred in Allentown and Billiers is in fact typical of national mental health policy patterns in the United States and France, respectively. The supply of US psychiatric care is so limited that only a small portion of the 50 million Americans who have a mental illness obtain treatment for it (Kohn et al. 2018; NIMH 2021). France,

---

(*Lehighvalleylive.com*), February 22, 2010; Bernie O'Hare, "Local Unions to Rally Tomorrow against Closing Allentown State Hospital," *Lehigh Valley Ramblings* (blog), February 1, 2010; "Billiers. Les salariés du centre de réadaptation inquiets," *Ouest-France*, September 29, 2015; "Centre de Postcure de Billiers. Manifs ce matin et cet après-midi," *Le Télégramme*, October 13, 2015; CFDT CPR de Billiers, "Sauvons le CPR de Billiers," 2015; "Decision to Shut Allentown Facility Final; About 55 Patients Heading to Wernersville State Hospital," *The Reading Eagle*, February 24, 2010; "Department of Public Welfare to Close Allentown State Hospital," *The Express-Times* (*Lehighvalleylive.com*), January 28, 2010; "Domaine de Prières. Forte mobilisation," *Le Télégramme*, October 14, 2015; Jacqueline Palochko, "'Give It a New Life': Small Group Protests Demolition of Allentown State Hospital," *The Morning Call*, October 26, 2019; Kurt Bresswein, "Fate of Allentown State Hospital Is in Lawmakers' Hands," *The Express-Times* (*Lehighvalleylive.com*), June 4, 2019; Pennsylvania Department of Public Welfare, "Allentown State Hospital Closure: Frequently Asked Question," 2010; "Santé. Les élus se mobilisent pour 'Sauver le CPR de Billiers,'" *Ouest-France*, October 6, 2015; "Sauvons le Centre de Réadaptation et de Postcure de Billiers," *Ouest-France*, September 10, 2015.

[4] The term "welfare state" refers to those public policies that protect individuals against the social risks incurred by market capitalism (following the classic definitions in, for instance, Baldwin 1992; Esping-Andersen 1990). Examples include health, social care, and income replacement policies (e.g., disability, pensions, unemployment insurance). Marginalized people such as those with severe mental illness are among those most at risk, for they are already disadvantaged in terms of their access to the labor market relative to regular wage-earners.

meanwhile, supplies more than double the care of its counterpart, facing fewer problems of shortage. But a mid 20th-century observer could not have predicted that the supply of public mental health services in France would eventually triple that of the United States. If anything, the opposite might have been more likely, as supply in France had degenerated and declined during the Second World War.

What is more, the cross-national differences in mental health care do not necessarily map onto the general trends in social welfare provision across countries. The large public welfare states of Norway and Sweden, for example, diverge on mental health care. More generally, these cross-national differences exist despite each of these countries' efforts to "de-institutionalize" patients. A process that began after the Second World War but which peaked in the 1970s and 1980s, deinstitutionalization sought to depopulate mental asylums and, social reformers promised, replace them with non-hospital, "community-based" alternatives. A range of factors contributed to this process, including postwar political enthusiasm for social reform, academic critiques of large mental institutions, and the rise of a film industry that spread these critiques into popular culture.[5] This international impetus, though, did not produce identical outcomes in domestic policy. To understand why, this book presents a comparative and historical analysis of mental health care development prior to and during deinstitutionalization (from the mid 19th to late 20th centuries) in the four countries mentioned, selected for their ability to inform broader trends in mental health services provision across the affluent democracies (where the deinstitutionalization movement first took root).[6] I draw on rich and often unexplored archival sources to explain the political origins of contemporary mental health care systems.

This book points to the central role of workers employed by the welfare state – what I call the "welfare workforce" – in shaping the supply of social services. These workers, an important segment of postindustrial labor markets and the linchpin of the contemporary trade union

---

[5] See, for example, Goffman (1961) or Szasz (1961), as well as *The Snake Pit* (1948) and *One Flew Over the Cuckoo's Nest* (1975), films based on novels by Ward (1946) and Kesey (1962), respectively.

[6] This term, "affluent democracies," will refer to the universe of cases to which this study primarily applies, which are also known as the advanced capitalist democracies. They are mostly found in Western Europe and Northern America, as well as English-speaking Oceania and parts of East Asia. Occasionally, I use the adjectives "postindustrial," "service-based," and/or "knowledge-based" to characterize the economic and labor market structure of these societies, which have shifted away from a dependence on industrial, especially manufacturing, employment and toward one of service employment instead.

movement, can become the most ardent defenders of their source of employment and, by extension, of services for the vulnerable. Most often employed in the public sector, they encompass a wide range of occupations and can include, for example, nurses, teachers, caregivers, facility support staff, and, importantly, managers. Absent powerful beneficiaries, the scope of public social services depends on the political influence of these workers' trade unions.

Yet they do not always succeed; their success can depend on whether managers participate in this advocacy, a unique source of political power for the public sector workforce. Like private sector managers, public sector managers can access the levers that change production capacities and alter compensation; however, they often happen to benefit from the same pay and protections as their subordinates. In short, public sector managers can make policy decisions that jointly benefit themselves and their employees. A coalition between these two groups within the welfare workforce can expand employment and service provision. Its absence, though, can reduce them. I find that a public labor–management coalition is more likely when public sector managers organize independently of private sector managers. This arrangement amplifies the political voice of public sector managers and facilitates their alliance with their employees. Such was the case in the development of French and Norwegian mental health policy, in contrast to that of the United States and Sweden, where the absence of a public labor–management coalition enabled the reduction of public mental health services.

To elaborate on this argument and the objectives of this book, this introductory chapter unfolds in three parts. First, it explains the importance of studying the field of mental health with the tools of comparative political economy; doing so can illuminate both areas. Herein the phrase "political economy" refers to the relationship between governments and markets, where the adjective "comparative" refers to how this relationship varies across countries. Although I use the term "mental health" to refer to all conditions requiring psychiatric or psychological care, I focus in particular on the most challenging and severe conditions that consume most of the public mental health system's resources (e.g., schizophrenia, chronic depression, severe bipolar disorder, and other severe mental illnesses). This first section also presents the theoretical puzzle and empirical questions of this book in greater detail. Second, it turns to the argument, providing more information about its logical coherence. Third, the chapter closes by articulating the research design and how it structures this book.

WHY STUDY THE COMPARATIVE POLITICAL ECONOMY OF MENTAL HEALTH?

Comparative political economists have spent very little time thinking about mental health policy, and mental health specialists have spent very little time thinking about comparative political economy. This has produced deficiencies in both areas. More fundamentally, the absence of engagement across these two fields is a disservice to the millions of people who experience a psychiatric condition. Neuropsychiatric conditions account for almost 30 percent of the global burden of disease in the affluent democracies, and as data collection improves, a growing percentage worldwide (WHO 2011). Despite these high needs, it can be difficult to finance, deliver, and sustain comprehensive and ample psychiatric services.

Often, in the minds of both the public and numerous scholarly observers, the challenges of mental health care delivery are the result of cultural, not political or economic, factors. Stigma, in particular, is often blamed (*The Lancet* 2016). But where does this stigma come from? It is partly the result of psychiatry's institutional heritage. Popular perceptions of insane asylums equated those buildings with social deviance, insofar as they relegated people with mental illness to a life of permanent seclusion. Eventually, so the story goes, a changing society opted to embrace the mentally ill, cease their confinement, and close the asylums. Yet the public could not completely decouple mental illness from its historical stigmatization, whose cultural legacy continues to plague policy today.

In one of the only political-economic studies of post-asylum mental health care, Andrew Scull (1984) questions this cultural narrative by tracing the structural development of psychiatric deinstitutionalization. Studying the examples of the United States and England, he demonstrates how the economic prosperity of the postwar period reduced the population of long-term residents in psychiatric hospitals, in part because the expanding welfare state created new social programs that made life outside the hospital more feasible for people with mental illness than it had been in the past. Rather than seek custodial and medical care in charitable institutions, patients could rely on increased access to disability benefits, health insurance, and public housing for support. What ultimately closed the asylums, Scull argues, was the advent of economic crisis in the 1970s. The welfare state had to make choices about which programs to keep and which to cut. The expensive mental institutions, whose resident patients had largely left, were first on the chopping block. Although

mental health reformers had hoped to replace these hospitals with outpatient and non-hospital alternatives, these countries lacked the political
and financial will to do so. The result was a failed policy transition, as
well as the continued relegation of the mentally ill to the unattended, stig-
matized corners of society.

Scull's compelling analysis has contributed to the centrality of the
Anglo-American, and especially the US, experience in the structural
interpretations of psychiatric deinstitutionalization (see also Brown
1985; Dear and Wolch 1987; Jones 1993; Rochefort 1993). The term
"de-institutionalization" has in fact become the anglicism imported by
non-English speaking scholars to describe that process in their home
countries, even though alternative language might be more context-
appropriate (e.g., the French "*déshopitalisation*," Coldefy 2010; see also
Chapireau 2021). The international literature often presumes that this
process will result in institutional closures, as was the case with American
state and county mental hospitals. It also assumes that countries will
struggle to provide outpatient and non-hospital services, as was the case
with the US community mental health center program (WHO 2014a).

Ironically, comparative and historical political-economic research was
foundational to the study of the welfare state even while mental health
has thus far been excluded from this work. Perhaps that Anglo-American
focus is one of the reasons why. Not only has much welfare state research
focused on the (non-Anglo) European cases, the existing (US-inflected)
interpretation of psychiatric deinstitutionalization in many ways conforms with how scholars of the American politics subfield understand the
development of US social policy. While at one point the United States did
provide some substantial welfare benefits, they soon became associated
with unequal 19th-century systems of patronage, perceived as a threat to
the country's racialized economy and geography, or otherwise encountered too many political hurdles in the country's veto-ridden federal, congressional, presidential, and judicial system (Lieberman 1998; Mettler
1998; Skocpol 1992; Weir et al. 1988). Asylums, in short, were bound
to close in the United States. Even if they did make it past the 19th and
early 20th centuries, these hospitals would face steep opposition from the
politicians attempting to retrench and/or privatize social benefits in the
late 20th century (Hacker 2002; King 1987; Pierson 1994). More generally, the United States' limited welfare state prefers to distribute benefits
to (white) recipients whose hard work has rendered them "deserving"
(Gilens 1999; Quadagno 1994), a designation the destitute mentally ill
could not hope to achieve.

For comparative political economists, the presumed lack of financial importance of the mental health care sector has put it in a secondary position relative to the big-budget items of the welfare state, such as pensions, education, and general health care. Nor is mental health care clearly tied to the labor market and its needs, precisely the area that the welfare state seeks to redress. Moreover, the Anglo-American experience of psychiatric deinstitutionalization also conforms with how scholars of comparative politics understand the national types of social policy (Goodwin 1997). That the United States and England were unable to maintain and expand mental health care after deinstitutionalization may not be very surprising, given that these countries belong to the "liberal" category of welfare states (Esping-Andersen 1990) and the "liberal" variety of capitalism (Hall and Soskice 2001). In these contexts, the state is much less likely to intervene in the market and provide social benefits to workers than it is in Scandinavia and continental Europe, the home of the "social democratic" and "corporatist" categories of welfare states and the "coordinated" variety of capitalism.

And yet some countries *do* devote significant public resources to the nonworking mentally ill. They also manage to provide extensive outpatient – and inpatient – care. These cross-national variations, furthermore, do not map onto the typologies of welfare states or capitalism that anchor comparative political economy. Figure 1.1 plots the supply of psychiatric care across 16 affluent democracies. These countries were the first to experience deinstitutionalization, since their early industrialization in the 19th century prompted the rise of the asylum, while their economic prosperity in the 20th century prompted its decline. Contrary to the presumed logic of deinstitutionalization described above, the countries that maintained more hospital care (or "institutional" care, which Figure 1.1 measures in terms of psychiatric beds) also tended to expand more non-hospital care (or "community" care, which Figure 1.1 measures in terms of outpatient and nonresidential facilities). Those countries also tend to spend more public resources on mental health care. Although the anglophone cases tend to fall at the lower end of the supply spectrum, they are not alone there. Social democratic and corporatist welfare states, such as Sweden, Denmark, Italy, and Austria, also provide low levels of inpatient and outpatient mental health care. Meanwhile, other countries with coordinated market economies provide starkly different distributions of care. In short, the supply of public mental health services varies across the affluent democracies, in ways not expected by either mental health scholars or comparative political economists.

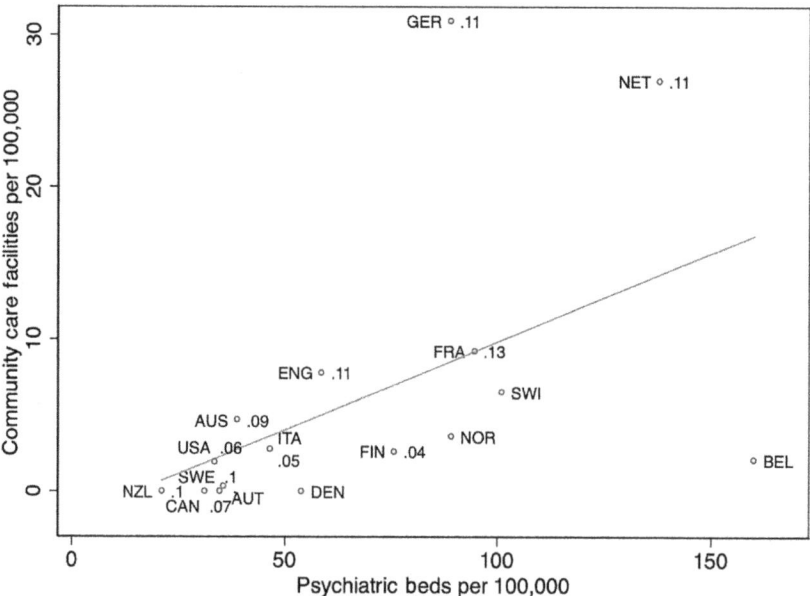

FIGURE 1.1 Scatterplot of psychiatric beds and community care facilities per 100,000 in 16 high-income democracies, with percentage of health budget allocated to mental health (as available) and line of best fit
Source: WHO (2011)

These variations do not map onto the expected national typologies of welfare states and capitalisms in part because those models presumed a very different economy, one based on industrial and, especially, manufacturing labor. Although scholars have observed that these models may not fully represent the approaches of contemporary governments to the postindustrial, liberalized, service-based, and knowledge economy (e.g., Baccaro and Howell 2017; Pierson 2001), less has been made of the fact that services now occupy a staggering segment of the welfare state itself. Models of welfare states center on the primary role of social transfers – such as pensions, unemployment insurance, and health insurance – in compensating formal, industrial, and largely male workers. Heroic efforts have certainly been made to characterize the scale and scope of the rising social service sectors in the welfare state, areas that include the development of secondary and tertiary educational institutions, advanced and more complex health care services, and long-term care services for children, the elderly, and the disabled (Alber 1995; Castles 2009; Jensen 2008, 2011). Since scholars must develop specialized expertise to understand each of these social service sectors, they are often studied in isolation.[7] Attempts to examine them together or to generalize across sectors are less common.

Much can be gained by analyzing the comparative politics of social service provision in the postindustrial economy as a comprehensive trend. In one important study, *Making Markets in the Welfare State* (2011), Jane Gingrich examines why policy-makers have recently adopted different approaches to marketizing social services, finding that the interests of service providers play a crucial role in the outcomes chosen by politicians. In cases of large-scale or universal social services, such as the entire education or health care sector, Gingrich argues that the preferences of a broad client group can motivate politicians to introduce market mechanisms to improve service quality, delivery, or distribution. Whether and how politicians act, though, depends both on their partisan orientation and on how the preexisting structure of the social service shapes provider interests. According to Gingrich, the interaction of partisan and provider preferences, in turn, shapes the type of market reform pursued.

Building on where Gingrich left off, this study develops the political economy that sustains services for the disenfranchised, a group of pressing concern in an era of sharp political, social, and economic inequalities. In fact, even the studies of social services in developing countries can presume some client demand, insofar as politicians deploy those services as instruments of patronage and vote-buying (e.g., Auerbach 2019; Stokes 2013; Thachil 2014; Wilfahrt 2022). But unlike the mobilized constituencies invested in protecting large-scale and universal social services, services such as mental health care, elderly care homes, or schooling for poor children lack this political pressure.[8] The same issue arises

---

[7] In fact, the American Political Science Association has developed specialized sections on health and education politics, respectively. This book, with its niche focus on mental health care, cannot claim to absolve itself of that pattern of specialization, but only to develop a theoretical framework applicable across multiple social service areas.

[8] Gingrich (2011) includes an analysis of marketization in the elderly care sector alongside that of large-scale reforms in health and education. She finds that electoral constraints play a smaller role (and public sector unions can play a larger one) in elderly care sector than in others, in part because of its residual nature. Worth noting is its distinctly complex client base. On the one hand, middle-class working-age adults may advocate for more assistance caring for their older parents and organized pensioners may value that support. On the other hand, these groups may be willing to accept (even prefer) some private provision of these services, and the issue may not be central to their vote choice. Moreover, the clients in greatest need of these services – the destitute elderly – tend to lack political representation. Indeed, Morgan and Campbell (2005) have shown how the political economy of the elderly care sector shares similarities with both those studied by

for social services delivered to noncitizens, such as undocumented immigrants, or in democratically unincorporated regions, such as the overseas territories of many of the affluent democracies.

Mental health care, then, is a window into the political economy of social service provision to disenfranchised and destitute populations, who lack the electoral power to motivate politicians to reform or expand those services. Although mental health has recently entered popular conversations about personal well-being, sustained mobilization tends to be limited to the efforts of a few families. This is a political constituency that is often geographically dispersed (and less compelling to elected officials), usually middle class or affluent (and able to share some of the costs of care with government), and primarily concerned with intellectual and developmental conditions (not those of poorer adults with severe and chronic illness). These important efforts notwithstanding, beneficiary advocacy is much less common in mental health than in some other social policy areas, and with good reason.

Consider the experience of schizophrenia. Prevalence rates cut across national boundaries in ways that are broadly comparable (Charlson et al. 2018). This severe mental illness can inhibit the basic activities of daily life, such as doing household chores or paying the bills, and so the act of political organization becomes even less likely. Moreover, the condition tends to present itself in early adulthood, often after completing compulsory education but before obtaining occupational security. This unfortunate timing reduces the incentives for either the educational system or the labor market to address the condition. Nor does this timing enable people with schizophrenia to access work-based social benefits or accrue the necessary disposable income to demand services with the help of their unions, wallets, or, for that matter, political parties. Where schizophrenia and other forms of serious mental illness contain socially constructed components, furthermore, they do so in ways that align with a society's existing axes of marginality and political impoverishment (see, for example, Metzl 2009). In exacerbating these vulnerabilities, mental illness is an extreme example of weak demand, thereby shifting and focusing political analysis squarely on the supply side.

Gingrich and those I explore here. Examining the politics of long-term care in Germany and the United States, they point to the role of local elected officials. Representing both their local (under-mobilized) constituents and their state government's budgetary needs, these political actors advocated for resource expansion. An institutional factor, the structure of federalism in each country, allowed German representatives to be more successful than their American counterparts.

Beyond its ability to explain the distribution of welfare to the disenfranchised, a study of mental health care can also inform studies of public services more generally for two reasons. First is its "public" component; that is, its heavy dependence on government financing. For the reasons discussed above, very few clients can afford to pay for costly, labor-intensive psychiatric services on their own. Consider how the unadjusted costs of psychotherapy could amount to a patient's monthly rent or more. If a licensed professional therapist earns $100–$200 per hour of treatment, weekly meetings (the usual clinical recommendation) would amount to $400–$800. Government subsidies of those labor costs hence reduce those high out-of-pocket costs for clients.

Mental health services that cannot rely on public funding reduce their size and scope, relying instead on patients with resources to sustain less-intensive services. The provision of mental health care, as a result, can be especially unequal, since recipients are either unable to afford costly long-term treatments (and therefore depend on public generosity) or are sufficiently moneyed to cover the substantial out-of-pocket health and social care costs associated with mental illness (see Perera 2019). Providers tend to serve one clientele or the other, with higher needs among the former group. The lines between public and private care have become increasingly blurred, particularly as welfare states continue to delegate provision to the private market and introduce market reforms to public services and policies (Gingrich 2011; Mettler 2011; Morgan and Campbell 2011); but even services that delegate mental health provision to private actors still tend to rely on public financing to support it.

Second is the "services" component of mental health care. In addition to depending heavily on public financing, mental health care includes components from all three core social services: education, health, and care. Since its inception in the 19th century, mental health care has stood out for its combination of medical and custodial care, financed, if not outright delivered, by government (see Ansell and Lindvall 2020). Over time, educational and vocational services have become part of the equation too, as society began to perceive the mentally ill as both capable, even desirous, of employment and schooling. Today, mental health care can involve a wide range of professionals, such as doctors, nurses, therapists, social workers, caregivers, vocational instructors, and special needs teachers, as well as the administrative and maintenance staff required to operate a variety of facilities.

Like other social services, mental health care has experienced significant pressures to reduce its labor-intensive costs. These strains became acute during the deinstitutionalization period, as Scull (1984) observed. The two most threatening factors to peak during this time were those that beset all services: automation and cost-control. When the first antipsychotic medication hit medical markets in the 1950s, it threatened to replace much of the work conducted by the staff of mental health institutions. As an automatic sedative, it reduced the amount of time that staff spent constraining patients who were experiencing difficult episodes, as well as that spent engaging them in other activities to avoid relapses. By the time the economic crisis hit in the 1970s, governments (urged by pharmaceutical companies) had realized that patients could take these medications on their own, outside of the expensive hospital system and with the help of the expanded "outdoor relief" of the postwar welfare state. The state pressure to reduce costs and close down hospitals became a ubiquitous force across the affluent democracies. Moreover, these pressures increased over the subsequent decades, as attempts to privatize, marketize, or otherwise retrench public services accelerated. The fact that some countries retained and even expanded their supply of public mental health care suggests that politics can help to explain why some services resist these pressures.

In sum, a study of the comparative political economy of mental health, in historical perspective, is instructive for several reasons. First, mental health specialists lack an explanation for why the supply of mental health care varies across countries, which is attributable neither to cultural factors (as a political economy perspective has already shown) or to a single, unifying set of conditions (to date, the dominant way of understanding the structural dynamics of mental health care provision). Second, the cross-national differences in supply suggest that sometimes welfare states deliver social services to clients who are unable to demand them. These differences bring to light a puzzle whose solution has become even more necessary in recent decades, as inequality increases and services (especially public social services) expand in the affluent democracies. Not only is demand for mental health care especially weak, the challenges in its provision are emblematic of all public services. Despite their heavy dependence on government financing and significant cost pressures, public mental health services have managed to survive, and even thrive, in some countries. The theoretical contribution of this book is to explain why, as detailed in the remainder of this chapter.

THE WELFARE WORKFORCE AND SUPPLY-SIDE
POLICY FEEDBACK: A THEORY OF ALLIANCES

The politics of the "welfare workforce" can explain why the supply of mental health services diverges across countries and, indeed more generally, why the supply of public social services for the disenfranchised often varies as well. When services lack robust demand, their maintenance and expansion can hang on those who depend on them for their employment. Public service employees have become a significant segment of the labor force in affluent democracies, on average one of every five workers is now employed by the state, most often in the health, education, and care sectors (OECD 2021). As employees of the welfare state, these workers have a strong interest in maintaining and expanding its public social service infrastructure. Otherwise they might lose their jobs, which are among the best compensated and protected in postindustrial, and increasingly precarious, economies.

Although the welfare workforce can play a role across the gamut of social services, it is especially influential for services with weak client demand. As Gingrich (2011) has demonstrated, the distribution of social services with broad, universal support depends on the relationships between constituents, partisan politicians, and providers. My research builds on that work, exploring the provision of social services that lack such electoral support. Without mobilized beneficiaries and, by extension, the politicians that represent them, providers become the key political stakeholder. But providers do not always succeed in maintaining and expanding the welfare state.

Figure 1.2 illustrates the theory of "supply-side policy feedback," which I have developed to explain when, why, and how welfare state employees can alter the course of social policy. This term draws on the scholarly literature in American political science on "policy feedback," which demonstrates how the structure of public policy conditions elite and public demand for it, in turn reinforcing that structure (Campbell 2003; Mettler and Soss 2004; Patashnik 2008; Weir and Skocpol 1985).[9] The politics of services for the disenfranchised, though, can depend more on the politics of supply than those of demand. In *supply-side* policy feedback, the structure of public policy conditions *suppliers'* demand for it, producing a similar, self-reinforcing pattern. Unlike theories of policy feedback that focus on

---

[9] In this way, this study contributes to calls and efforts to extend policy feedback theory across a wider set of country cases beyond the United States (see Béland and Schlager 2019; Busemeyer et al. 2021; Bussi et al. 2022; Gingrich and Watson 2016).

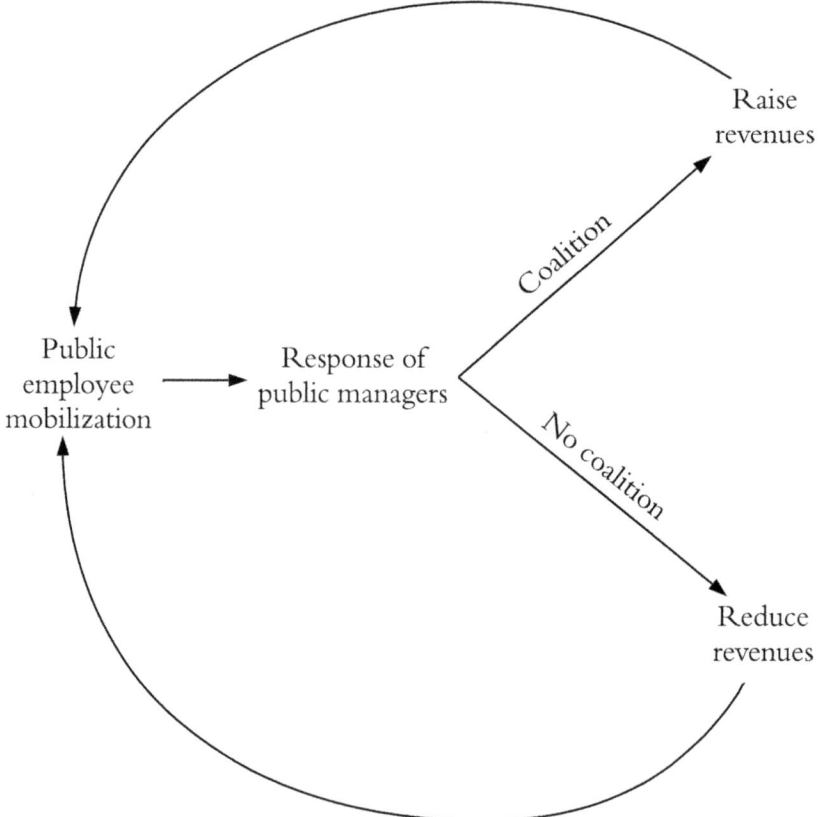

Positive feedback:
more public services, employment security and
protections, workforce growth, support for labor rights

Negative feedback:
fewer public services, reduced wages and
protections, layoffs, less support for labor rights

FIGURE 1.2 Supply-side policy feedback model: Effects of public sector worker alliances on the supply of public social services for disenfranchised populations (basic diagram of theoretical argument)

elite and mass politics, this theory emphasizes the meso-level: the role of workers who depend on those policies for their employment (the welfare workforce).

The supply-side policy feedback process begins when services face sharp cost-containment pressure, pushing the wages of employees downward. Cost pressures are formidable and frequent in these service sectors. For example, related or automated services can become serious competitors. Nor are the growing service sectors able to compete with wage increases in the smaller but more productive sectors, such as manufacturing (Baumol and Bowen 1966). Public services are also subject to political deregulation and government cost-containment initiatives.[10] Each of these factors incentivize service providers to reduce costs, especially in their most expensive budget line: labor and wages.

In response to these cost pressures and downward wage pressures, the employees of these services mobilize, so long as public policies, laws, and regulations permit them to do so. Where organized labor can strike, bargain, and advocate for its interests, workers can mobilize to preserve their employment, resist layoffs, and advocate for wage increases. Institutional context, whether national or occupational, is important. Compare, for instance, teachers and caregivers. Differences in the organizational rights and capacities afforded to each group, as well as the public or private sector location of their employment, have granted them very different degrees of political voice. While protests by public sector teachers' unions have become a fixture of the postindustrial economy, the same cannot be said for private caregivers. Whether and how workers mobilize, then, is the second step of the supply-side policy feedback process.

The third step can be the most consequential for the fate of public services. Here workers can develop the political alliances necessary to procure protection and compensation. Sometimes, politicians can become important allies of public service employees (Anzia and Moe 2016). A particular district's or party's dependence on public employment, for instance, can incentivize elected officials to respond to their demands. But note that this theory departs from others developed on public sector employees by focusing on their role as workers, not voters. In cases where clients are disenfranchised and the electoral relevance of the policy area is low, public sector trade unions seeking to protect the employment of their members might turn to actors other than politicians for support, such as interest groups, professional associations, and even sympathetic social movements.

Of particular importance to this theory, therefore, is the presence or absence of a political alliance between public service managers and public

---

[10] As proposed in other work with Brown (Perera and Brown, in press), "public" services are those that receive a sizeable share of their revenue from the state and, crucially, are owned and operated by national and local governments. Meanwhile, "private" services receive most, if not all, of their revenue from the private sector and are private legal entities.

service workers. To be sure, it can be difficult to define "managers" and "workers" in the public sector. A distal and complex principal–agent relationship characterizes public sector labor relations, especially given the role of elected officials as potential principals (Moe 2006). State-employed managers, this theory underscores, are another set of principals. I hence define public managers as those government-employed supervisors whose positions do not depend on electoral politics and political appointments. Public managers nonetheless may make decisions about hiring and firing, workplace protections, and production capacities (like their counterparts in the private sector); but they do not "own" the means of production (unlike those counterparts). Rather, public managers remain dependent on government funds and employment contracts for their wages. They can include the heads of government schools, the directors of public hospitals, or the administrators of public childcare services. Public workers are their supervisees, who also depend on government funds and employment contracts for their wages.[11]

Unlike labor–management relations in the private sector, in the public sector these relations are not necessarily antagonistic. In the private sector, managers are often responsible for maximizing revenue while minimizing labor costs, incentives that tend to put them at odds with rank-and-file workers, who would, on average, prefer higher compensation and strong job protections. But because many of the incentives private sector managers face are often relaxed in the public sector – managers, for example, are rarely concerned with profit margins – managers and workers are often much less at odds. For example, managers' employment contracts and benefit packages are often very close, if not identical, to those of their own employees. Perhaps more importantly, the two ultimately have a shared interest in protecting their source of employment, especially when proposals that introduce high levels of insecurity, such as those to cut funding or privatize the existing institution, emerge. Cross-class coalitions can therefore be more common in the public sector than the private sector because workers and managers have stronger incentives to align.

---

[11] Although the relationship between workers and managers is particularly complicated in the public sector, both the increasing stratification of workers and the service transition have challenged it in the private sector, too. Moreover, workers and managers in the private sector sometimes organize together, too. See, for example, Gourevitch and Shinn (2007), as well as the scholarship documenting when and why business elites support redistributive and compensatory policies for their employees (Mares 2003; Martin and Swank 2012; Swenson 2002).

When the state threatens to reduce the supply of public services, employees mobilize using the usual tools of labor influence, such as strike action. In doing so, they generate pressure that urges managers to respond. One way to raise funds is to charge clients more for services, but this approach is unreliable if clients are poor. Instead, and following Niskanen's (1971) classic formulation, public managers can become "budget maximizers" who can turn to the state to obtain secure and generous compensation for public services. Departing from Niskanen, though, I propose that what motivates managers to do so is the strong pressure of their employees, for labor costs are often the largest line item of most public budgets.[12] Public managers are unlikely to advocate without this employee pressure, especially since managers tend to have more opportunities to exit to private industry when their public sector careers are no longer viable.

This alliance shapes eventual policy choices through two main mechanisms. The first is "brokerage" – that is, when an individual or group connects previously disconnected social sites.[13] Acting as brokers between the public sector workforce and policy-makers, public sector managers can draw on the various tools at their disposal to shape public policy choices. Furthermore, the complex principal–agent relationships that characterize the public sector mean that "managers" can work at multiple levels of government and, by extension, control a broad range of rent-extracting tools. These efforts can reap considerable rewards for the coalition and the protection of public employment as a whole.

The second mechanism works through the "adaptive expectations" of policy-makers.[14] Simply put, policy-makers agree to increase funds in order to avoid escalating retribution from the powerful coalition. These sanctions can take multiple forms. For example, sustained labor unrest against cutbacks may pose a significant public disturbance, for which policy-makers may want to avoid any associated blame. Or politicians might worry that public sector workers will penalize them at the ballot box in their next term (as documented, for instance, by Anzia and Moe 2016). Electoral considerations can reenter the distributive equation here; but they might not. Exacerbating these potential penalties are

---

[12] Note, where labor is weak, the coalition can only procure some – but not substantial – revenue growth (compare the first and second feedback cycles discussed in Chapter 5).

[13] For a discussion of this mechanism, see McAdam et al. (2001); Falleti and Lynch (2009).

[14] For a discussion of this mechanism, see Pierson (2000a) (building on Arthur 1994); Falleti and Lynch (2009).

those techniques deployable by public managers. Stifling the progress of an important policy-making commission or refusing to administer a public service, for instance, can cause headaches for both elected and unelected officials. Policy-makers hence retract attempts to cut back on public funding after realizing the political costs of doing so.

Many factors can influence whether the public labor–management coalition can form, though in this book I primarily focus on one: the organizational structure of public managers. As I have argued elsewhere, how a group aggregates the interests of its members can shape its public policy agenda (Perera 2022).[15] Where a united group of public sector managers can express their interests independently of private sector managers, they are more likely to form a coalition with public sector workers. Organizations that independently represent public managers have clear economic priorities, advocating only on behalf of the public sector. Organizations that represent both public and private managers, however, must contend with the competing positions of each camp. An organization with a mixed attitude hence is unlikely to become a strong promoter of public services. Moreover, it is important that public managers speak with a single voice. A singular focus on the public sector also makes public managers facing a hostile bargaining environment both more willing and more effective, especially when urged to do so by employee allies. It also encourages cohesion between different types of public managers (e.g., at varying levels of government or service areas). Where the political representation of public managers is fragmented, they are likely to express differing policy agendas. Those conflicts can make it difficult to solidify an alliance with workers. Public managers who organize together and independently of their private sector counterparts, therefore, are better equipped to satisfy workers' demands to raise revenues, form a political coalition, and help to increase the supply of public services for the beneficiaries who cannot demand them.

This public labor–management coalition is therefore a unique source of political power for state employees and can have long-lasting effects on social service provision. When stable and regular, these otherwise strange bedfellows can procure generous revenues and protections from

---

[15] This argument build on a tradition of similar arguments made about trade unions, business organizations, and grassroots activists, which point to the political repercussions of organizational structure and institutional rules on preference expression (Ahlquist and Levi 2013; Anderson and Lynch 2007; Collier and Handlin 2009; Frymer 2005; Golden 1993; Han 2014; Levi et al. 2009; Nijhuis 2013; Oliver 2011; Schmitter and Streeck 1999).

government, reinforcing the political strength of the welfare workforce, spurring additional rounds of policy feedback, and expanding public social services. The absence of a durable coalition has the opposite effect: Without the political alliance with management, public sector workers can have difficulty procuring support from government, which results in less revenue, fewer protections, and the retrenchment of public services. These patterns produce what policy feedback scholars call "positive" and "negative" effects, respectively (see Jacobs and Weaver 2015; Pierson 2000b; Weaver 2010).

These self-reinforcing feedback effects notwithstanding, the public labor–management coalition holds independent influence on policy outcomes. Without it, the initial cycle cannot launch. Although institutional factors may influence the propensity of the welfare workforce to form alliances, they do not necessarily determine them (nor do they independently predict the policy outcome, an alternative hypothesis discussed in Chapter 2). Although state actors may attempt to manipulate alliance formation, they are more likely to do so in subsequent feedback cycles, and usually only once the coalition has demonstrated its potency. Reversing the direction of feedback is nonetheless possible, particularly if the coalition is not yet very powerful nor very weak. More generally, the presence or absence of a public labor–management coalition prompts alternative path-dependent processes in which the alliance gradually gains or loses political power over time. These two supply-side policy feedback cycles have shaped the trajectory of mental health service provision across the West.

COMPARING MENTAL HEALTH CARE OVER TIME AND ACROSS COUNTRIES

Explaining why the supply of mental health care varies across countries requires analyzing the policies that structure those differences and how they developed over time. Structural outcomes such as public policies have multiple and complex causes. To isolate the most salient and determinative factors for mental health policy, I compare the late 20th-century process of psychiatric deinstitutionalization in two countries with similar initial conditions but different contemporary outcomes: the United States and France. To assess whether these factors can explain variation elsewhere, I then trace them in Sweden and Norway, a concise comparison that also allows me to rule out a few unresolved alternative hypotheses from the first comparison.

Explaining highly aggregated outcomes such as mental health policies requires thorough attention to both their individual parts and their systematic whole. The analytic approach of this book is therefore comparative, historical, and political-economic, examining how the relationship between politics and markets evolves over time and across governments. It takes into account how economic and political incentives combine to shape structural outcomes, such as those of an entire public policy area or economic sector. A historical perspective allows exploring the complete range of potential causal factors, including the chain of events that shaped their evolution. A comparative perspective, in turn, helps to narrow the list of potential causes by evaluating patterns in their presence or absence across cases. In this way, a cause that may seem important to one case is subject to testing and confirmation in another. This approach hence guides the analysis toward identifying the most important factors driving complex outcomes in contemporary political economies.

To help identify cases for comparison, the study begins by systematically charting the variation in public mental health care provision across affluent democracies and over time (this is developed in more detail in Chapter 2). To date, most of the research on mental health care provision has tended to examine individual countries, without a clear sense of how it compares to that of other countries (for an exception, see Goodwin 1997). Much of this predicament is due to the inherent difficulty of comparing indicators across national contexts, as they are often collected and defined in very different ways. A recent data collection initiative of the World Health Organization, however, aims to redress this problem. I use this standardized data to analyze contemporary differences in mental health care supply in the affluent democracies, the countries that first pursued deinstitutionalization reforms and set global expectations for public policy in this area (Figure 1.1). I also explore whether and how the historical evolution of mental health care supply may have shaped these differences, using the novel data set described in the Appendix. That effort reviewed the national statistical yearbooks of the 16 countries where deinstitutionalization first took root, collected data on mental health care services over the full course of deinstitutionalization, as well as tracked the initial conditions of supply, how it changed during that international wave, and with what results for 21st-century mental health systems (1935–2000). The data shows that all countries experienced deinstitutionalization but to widely varying degrees.

Drawing on the guidelines for case selection in comparative politics, I select two major countries where deinstitutionalization produced contrasting outcomes, despite the presence of important similarities prior to its onset. For this purpose, I select the United States, as noted the most influential case in the scholarly literature on deinstitutionalization, and France, of which relatively little has been written (especially in English). The two countries shared similar mental health and social care systems prior to deinstitutionalization. Policy-makers in both countries adopted similar blueprints to reform mental health care in the postwar period, notably with better prospects for implementation in the United States than in France. But the two systems eventually diverged.[16] I trace three supply-side policy feedback loops in each case, from the 1960s to the 1980s, documenting how the presence or absence of cross-class coalitions in the public sector shaped the increase of services in France and their decrease in the United States.

Although this paired historical comparison is able to eliminate a wide range of general and case-specific alternative hypotheses, it is nonetheless important to assess the validity of these findings in other countries. Because of the complex and context-specific knowledge required to analyze mental health care systems and their development, I have undertaken a second paired comparison of two smaller countries (instead of a "large-N" statistical analysis of far more governments, where this complexity could be lost). For this purpose, I selected Sweden and Norway, two expansive Nordic welfare states with uncharacteristically different approaches to mental health care. As Ansell and Lindvall (2020) note, Sweden, like the United States, had high rates of psychiatric institutionalization in the 1930s (over 0.3 percent, Ansell and Lindvall 2020), but rates fell dramatically later in the 20th century. This trend stands in contrast to what occurred in France and Norway. Moreover, and mirroring the contrasting patterns in the United States and France, Sweden's lower mental health care supply has received more attention in the international literature on deinstitutionalization than Norway's much higher

---

[16] Setting the postwar period as the critical juncture helps to refute the methodological challenge of historical regress – that is, at what point in time did an outcome's "cause" really originate and, by extension, at what point in time should the analyst begin their controlled comparison (Pierson 2004)? Bolstering the periodization of this study is that (1) before the Second World War there were no major "critical antecedents" that predetermined the countries' eventually diverging policy outcomes (Slater and Simmons 2010) and (2) after the Second World War, policy-makers in both countries sought similar outcomes (but did not universally succeed). Furthermore, and following practical recommendations for research deploying Mill's methods in the social sciences, I select cases that control for or rule out major alternative hypotheses, including potentially confounding background conditions (Slater and Ziblatt 2013).

supply. I trace one supply-side policy feedback loop in each case, since their divergence occurred primarily in the last decade of the 20th century (when economic crisis prompted their governments to speed up deinstitutionalization, which like that of its counterparts in the United States and France had already begun during the postwar period of welfare state expansion).

Studying these four cases in comparative, historical, and political-economic perspective is not only substantively instructive; it also departs from conventional approaches to political science research. First, this perspective is rare in the study of American public policy and politics. The organization and development of the political science discipline has foreclosed opportunities to apply this lens to the United States, instead fostering research on the country's peculiar political institutions and the opinions and behavior of its citizens. These avenues have generated important contributions to US politics, and indeed (if unintentionally) elsewhere, where Americanist research is often influential. Much can be gained, however, by incorporating a comparative and historical political-economic lens, insofar as it can help identify possible oversights in the field to date. Pioneer research by a few Americanists – notably those who have tended to write on the intersection of social policy and American political development – have already demonstrated the utility of comparative and historical political-economic analysis for the study of the United States (e.g., King 1995; Pierson 1994; Sheingate 2001; Weir and Skocpol 1985). The study of US health politics, in particular, has benefited from a tradition of comparative research (e.g., Giaimo 2002; Gusmano et al. 2010; Jacobs 1993; Maioni 1998; Tuohy 2018). Such work has been foundational to the emerging sub-disciplinary field of American political economy (Hacker et al. 2021). This book builds on and advances this under-utilized lens in American politics research.

Incorporating non-European countries in this study (through a close case analysis of the United States and the inclusion of Australia, Canada, and New Zealand in quantitative, cross-national comparisons) also expands the conventional comparative-historical scholarship on social policy and political economy, where the experience of Western Europe has been the dominant focus. Although the landmark typologies of welfare states and capitalist varieties include the affluent democracies of Northern America, East Asia, and Oceania (Esping-Andersen 1990; Hall and Soskice 2001), only a few scholars have devoted substantial attention to those countries (e.g., Estévez-Abe 2008; Morgan 2006; Obinger et al. 2005; Pontusson 2005; Swenson 2002). This attention deficit is the result of both the regionalist structure of the political science discipline and the fact that most of the cases of interest are located in a single region. Here, too, an expanded case comparison can help to identify oversights. The political-economic development of the non-European cases often occurred later and under very different conditions (e.g., settler colonialism, internal racial division, Eastern business models) compared to Europe. Moreover, the peculiarities of the French case do not fit neatly into the existing typologies either (Schmidt 2003). France's presidential and republican (anti-monarchical) history, for example, breaks from the political patterns found in the parliamentary constitutional monarchies of its neighbors. Rich insights can emerge, therefore, from this French–American comparison, an unconventional one in political science (though for some examples of books on the politics of social policy that use this approach, see Morgan 2006; Toloudis 2012). Moreover, the inclusion of Sweden and Norway, whose levels of mental health care supply are respectively much lower and much higher than scholars might expect, offers a more nuanced take than the stylized facts about these countries.

The subsequent chapters present how supply-side policy feedback and public labor–management coalitions developed mental health policy, first with a detailed French–American comparison and then with a more concise Norwegian–Swedish comparison. As Chapter 3 describes, in the 19th century public managers in both the United States and France organized independently, but over time public managers in America allied with their private sector counterparts (in this case, academic neurologists and psychiatrists in private clinics) while French public managers maintained their separation and unity. This seemingly small organizational difference nonetheless had major implications for public mental health care workers during the period of psychiatric deinstitutionalization. American public sector workers had difficulty gaining the support of their managers, whose representatives privileged attention to private psychiatry, while in France the coalition between public workers and managers resisted attempts to retrench services during this time. Chapters 4 and 5 discuss the American and French postwar and late 20th-century pathways to deinstitutionalization, respectively, assessing relevant case-specific alternative explanations along the way, such as the role of the centralized state and generous welfare coverage in France or the role of federal-state politics and racialized, more limited, and privatized welfare coverage in the United States. Chapter 6 then assesses the validity of these findings in other countries by corroborating them in the abbreviated study of Norway and Sweden in the 1990s, ruling out the major remaining alternative hypotheses such

TABLE 1.1 *Independent and combined effects of the presence or absence of a public labor–management coalition on the expansion of public mental health services in four countries over time*

		Public managers join coalition	
		Yes	No
Public workers join coalition	Yes	France (post-1968), Norway (1990s): significant expansion	United States (post-1970s): no significant expansion
	No	France (pre-1968), United States (pre-1920s): no significant expansion	United States (1920s–1970s), Sweden (1990s, most reforms): no significant expansion

as the general strength of the public sector trade union movement or the influence of a state-oriented welfare state. None of these alternative hypotheses hold significant muster against the central hypothesis of this book: that an alliance between labor and management in the public sector, enabled by the independent and unified organization of public sector managers, granted the welfare workforce political influence over the maintenance and expansion of the service that employed them.

The four cases also work together to assess the argument in other ways. First, they allow me to leverage a range of historical moments to assess whether public mental health policy depends more on the support of public workers, public managers, or indeed their combined potency. Table 1.1 presents examples of what occurs under each of these scenarios, drawing on examples from throughout this book. This study finds that neither public workers alone nor public managers alone can resist retrenchment efforts. Second, the four cases can also test whether the argument travels across the main types of western welfare states and varieties of capitalism: the "liberal" anglophone countries of Europe, North America, and Oceania (exemplified here by the United States), as well as in the "coordinated" market economies of "conservative" continental Western Europe (here, France) and "social democratic" Nordic Europe (Norway and Sweden) (see Esping-Andersen 1990; Hall and Soskice 2001).

The empirical material for this study relies on a wide range of primary and secondary historical sources (the documents relevant to mental health policy-making prior to and during psychiatric deinstitutionalization), few of which have received much academic scrutiny to date. Prior to this study, many of the sources on mental health policy produced by professional and, especially, labor organizations (such as trade press, newsletters, and memoirs written by their leaders) had been under-utilized and under-analyzed. For example, Chapter 4 draws on the American Federation of State, County, and Municipal Workers' three expansive collections on psychiatric deinstitutionalization (45 linear feet, per RL PPAD),[17] an important source hitherto unexplored, to the best of my knowledge, by other scholars. In fact, across all four countries, extensive archival research brings a wealth of reports, administrative memoranda, meeting minutes, and newspaper clippings to scholarly attention. Bolstering these primary historical sources are out-of-print secondary sources consulted at national, industry, and medical research libraries. For supplementary information and when possible, I conducted interviews with key policy-makers and political actors. This book is distinctive, moreover, in that it discusses the material of several countries in English; to date very little has been written about the non-English speaking countries in English (especially France and Norway). The primary sources consulted are listed in the Bibliography and cited at a more detailed level in the chapters.

New sources bring new information to the study of mental health policy. In fact, they often draw out peripheral points made in other histories and bring them to the center of the analysis, producing an account that is historiographically distinct from others. Of particular note is this project's treatment of elite opinions. While Whiggish histories have tended to emphasize the idealistic intentions of mental health policy reformers (e.g., Barton 1987), critical histories, instead, note how medical superintendents and other powerful actors deployed mental health care and its institutions as instruments of social control (e.g., Rothman 1980).

I examine written documentation linking elites to politics to highlight how their political and institutional environment shaped their economic priorities. Although I pay particularly close attention to official organizational statements, following Swenson (2018) I also assess the completeness of these sources' claims by triangulating them, wherever possible, against those made elsewhere, such as commentary in flagship journals and trade press, testimonies at legislative hearings, and points of discussion in governmental meetings. Readers can assess my interpretations of these sources by consulting the detailed bibliographic information, and often the fully quoted material, in the text. Source triangulation therefore

---

[17] Archival sources are abbreviated in the chapters. For a guide to these abbreviations, please see the Bibliography.

allows me to develop a comprehensive understanding of various actors' demands, as well as whether and how their organizational representatives conveyed these demands to policy-makers. Taken as a whole, the sources consulted for this book shift attention away from elites' moral and therapeutic inclinations and toward the political, administrative, economic, and institutional incentives that may shape them.

Moving beyond the contributions and findings of this book, Chapter 7 concludes by advancing its implications for postindustrial welfare capitalism more broadly. Canonical theories explain the development and variation in welfare states by pointing to the role of left politicians and unionized private sector workers (Esping-Andersen 1990; Korpi 1983; Stephens 1979). This book, though, demonstrates that the rise of service employment, especially in the public sector, has shifted both the products and the politics of the welfare state. Today, social service administrators and unionized public service workers have decentered the influence of those conventional actors. A new political logic is motivating social policy. The conclusion explores that new logic, and its consequences for people with mental illnesses and other beneficiaries of social services.

2

Nowhere to Go?

The Supply of Mental Health Services across Countries

Observers of the American mental health system often lament that people seeking its help have "nowhere to go." Consider, for example, E. Fuller Torrey's influential 1988 book *Nowhere to Go: The Tragic Odyssey of the Homeless Mentally Ill*, or the more contemporary press attention given to the issue, such as the 2014 CBS *60 Minutes* report "Nowhere to Go: Mentally Ill Youth in Crisis" and the *USA Today* investigative piece "Cost of Not Caring: Nowhere to Go – the Financial and Human Toll for Neglecting the Mentally Ill" of the same year. The assumption I made that late Philadelphia evening I described in the Preface is, unfortunately, a nationwide reality.

Similar language is used in other countries. Note the title of a 2020 report from the Australian College of Emergency Medicine: "Nowhere Else to Go: Why Australia's Health System Results in People Getting 'Stuck' in Emergency Departments." Meanwhile, in the United Kingdom, a headline in *The Guardian* bemoans the absence of mental health services, reading: "'She Was Left with No One': How UK Mental Health Deteriorated during Covid." In Canada, the largest mental health and addiction teaching hospital, the Centre for Addiction and Mental Health, premiered the film *Nowhere to Go: A Brokered Dialogue* to raise awareness about the mental health issues faced by LGBTQ homeless youth. This observation – that mental health systems are too meager to attend to societal needs – seems universal.[1]

---

[1] Alex Abramovich, *Nowhere To Go: A Brokered Dialogue*, documentary collaboration with the Centre for Addiction and Mental Health, 2016; Liz Szabo, "Cost of Not Caring: Nowhere to Go – the Financial and Human Toll for Neglecting the Mentally Ill," *USA*

This chapter questions that claim. Previously unexplored international data shows that it is only in select societies – those that have had the greatest influence on scholarly perceptions of mental health care – that its users have nowhere to go. In many other countries, the supply of mental health care is much higher. Moreover, and contrary to the presumptions that guide global mental health care policy-making, these understudied countries provide both ample community care and ample inpatient care. The wide variation in the contemporary supply of mental health services across affluent democracies is surprising for several reasons. These differences align with neither the existing scholarly typologies of social policy systems nor those of health policy systems. Furthermore, these variations are present despite all countries' shared history of psychiatric deinstitutionalization, a process conceptualized and documented using an original historical data set. I then turn to proposing an explanation for these differences and developing an empirical strategy to assess it. I focus on the cases of the United States and France, along with Norway and Sweden, in order to control for a range of case-specific alternative hypotheses. The chapter concludes with brief descriptions of the mental health care systems in each of the four countries examined in this book.

CONTEMPORARY DIFFERENCES IN THE SUPPLY
OF MENTAL HEALTH CARE ACROSS COUNTRIES

Figure 2.1 plots the supply of mental health care across 16 affluent democracies. The data is drawn from the World Health Organization (WHO), which sends a standardized questionnaire to in-country experts, usually government officials, who submit national statistics on their mental health system according to set definitions. Although an incomplete reflection of case-specific particularities, the figure presents an adequate snapshot of general trends across countries, using the most recent year available (see Perera 2020c). The 16 countries included were the first in the world to deinstitutionalize, since their early industrialization prompted the rise of the asylum, and their postwar economic prosperity prompted its decline.[2] As a result, the shared experiences of

Today, May 12, 2014; Duggan et al. 2020; Sarah Johnson, "'She Was Left with No One': How UK Mental Health Deteriorated during Covid," *The Guardian,* September 21, 2020; Scott Pelley, "Nowhere to Go: Mentally Ill Youth in Crisis," CBS *60 Minutes,* January 26, 2014.
[2] For inclusion and exclusion criteria, please see the Appendix.

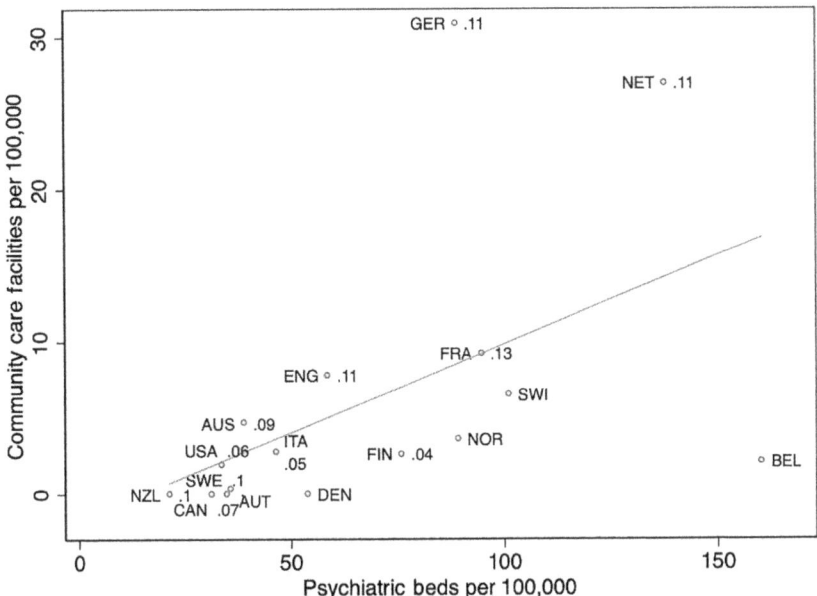

FIGURE 2.1 Scatterplot of psychiatric beds and community care facilities per 100,000 population in 16 high-income democracies and percentage of the public health budget spent on mental health (as available), with line of best fit
Source: WHO (2011)

these countries have framed global expectations in mental health, presuming that other countries will follow similar policy patterns as their economies develop.

Figure 2.1 reveals three important dimensions of variation in mental health care across countries. First, and despite the "nowhere to go" refrain, people with mental illnesses do have somewhere to go, in some countries. The supply of services in Germany, the Netherlands, Belgium, France, Switzerland, and Norway is much higher than in New Zealand, Canada, Sweden, Australia, Austria, the United States, and Italy. Second, the composition of services in the high-supply group includes both ample "institutional" care and ample "community" care. Institutional care, or hospital-based overnight care for people with mental disorders (operationalized in Figure 2.1 as psychiatric beds per 100,000) has gained a negative reputation among mental health specialists, who often view it as the outdated vestige of psychiatry's asylum period (WHO 2014a). They instead prefer community care, or non-hospital-based and outpatient care for people with mental disorders (operationalized as outpatient and day facilities per 100,000).[3] Nonetheless, countries with a generous supply of mental health care tend to include high amounts of both types of services. Moreover, countries at the higher end of the supply spectrum also tend to provide inpatient care in psychiatric hospitals, while those in the middle and at the lower end of the spectrum are more likely to deliver inpatient care in general hospitals (author's calculations using WHO 2011, not shown, see also Perera 2020a). In other words, countries that devote resources to separate psychiatric facilities appear to supply more inpatient care than those that do not. Third, the numbers to the right of each data point indicate, where available, the percentage of the government health budget allocated to mental health.[4] For the most part, countries that spend more of their public health budget on mental health tend to supply psychiatric care in greater quantities than those that do not.[5] This trend makes the mental health sector distinct from general health care, where the public sector accounts for far less of the supply of care (see also Perera 2019). Unlike general health services, mental health services are far more labor-intensive and serve more destitute clients, a combination of factors that renders mental health care costly and private investment unlikely.

These intertwined three dimensions of variation in mental health care systems therefore run counter to the presumptions that permeate global mental health policy paradigms. Consider the title of a press release from the Organisation for Economic Co-operation and Development (OECD): "The Netherlands has an innovative mental health system, but high bed

---

[3] The figure presents all available WHO data on mental health service provision in these countries, except for non-hospital residential facilities (present in only a few countries). These facilities blend elements of community and hospital services by combining non-medical social care with overnight care and cannot clearly be categorized as either community or inpatient care. Note also that the equivalent of "bed" data at the community level is not consistently available across countries, in part because capacity measures are less straightforward in outpatient facilities than they are in hospital facilities. Unlike hospitals that can provide overnight care in a discrete number of beds, community facilities may provide an adjustable range of services and activities throughout the day (e.g., the number of participants in a group therapy meeting might vary from week to week). For additional discussion of these data, see Perera (2020a, 2020c).

[4] An exception is the United States, which reported its mental health spending to the WHO as a percentage of overall (public and private) health care spending. Government expenditures alone are hence much lower in that country (about 60 percent of all mental health spending, see WHO 2011).

[5] Although the overall amount of the national public health budget can vary, measuring the percentage allocated to mental health care can describe the extent to which it is a policy priority, especially since mental health care necessarily requires more public financing than other areas of health care.

numbers remain a concern" (OECD 2014). The persistence of inpatient care, despite an otherwise admirable performance record, is presented as a paradox. Implied here is the notion that a modern, expansive psychiatric system should shrink the supply of inpatient care and replace it with outpatient care instead. Yet the largest mental health systems provide ample institutional care as well as community care. Contrary to international expectations, these two types of services appear to be complements, not substitutes (Perera 2020a). Their dependence on generous public financing, moreover, also challenges arguments that advocate for private investment in this policy area (Perera 2020b).

These three intertwined dimensions in fact are preconditions for a high-quality mental health system. Measuring the quality of mental health care is a notoriously challenging task (see the forum debates in *World Psychiatry* 2018). Much depends on the particular diagnosis of the user. For example, an adult experiencing clinical depression may require frequent access to a combination of psycho-therapeutic services and psycho-pharmaceuticals, provided in the daytime. Meanwhile, a child with autism might require pediatric behavioral and communication therapies. Other patients, such as those who experience psychotic episodes, may require periodic access to dignified overnight care. Complicating quality measurements further are the complex ethical issues that arise in mental health care. Patients do not always consent to receiving services, either because they do not believe they need them (a condition known as anosognosia) or simply because they are uncomfortable with what providers recommend. Moreover, what constitutes a "cure" in this area is often different than in general health care. Many conditions are chronic and recurring, such that successful service users often prefer to self-describe as "in recovery" rather than simply "recovered."

Nonetheless unifying these patient experiences is the need for widely available, comprehensive, and varied mental health care services, at low cost to the user. Experts agree that a "balanced" set of services ensures that all patients receive what they need, when they need it (Thornicroft and Tansella 2013). These services include those indicators captured in Figure 2.1: outpatient facilities where the patient experiencing clinical depression might obtain regular access to psychotherapy and pharmaceuticals, day care facilities where the child with autism might obtain psycho-pediatric services (and their parent might obtain relief from childcare responsibilities during the workday), and overnight inpatient services where the patient experiencing psychosis might obtain support for stabilization. Without these services, their conditions would remain untreated. Only an acute episode (e.g., a panic attack for the child, a suicide attempt for the adult with depression) would trigger contact with a hospital's stressful emergency department, hardly the site to relieve psychiatric trauma.

The public financing indicator in Figure 2.1 helps to capture how much these services cost their users. As I commented in *The Lancet Psychiatry* (2019), people with chronic behavioral health needs rarely have the means to afford their own care. Mental disability inhibits workforce entry, limiting the income available to cover private and out-of-pocket health care costs. Moreover, long-term mental health treatment requires different, often more complex resources than other health treatments (Franck and McGuire 2000). Public financing of these services is therefore common and necessary. Note that the public financing indicator normally excludes expenditures on psycho-pharmaceuticals. These drugs tend to be much cheaper to provide than labor-intensive care services, so governments tend to pay for them using standard pharmaceutical coverage schemes. More variable and often more consequential for users is whether and to what extent services are covered. When generously funded by the state, such services often result in low (or no) cost to users.

To be sure, Figure 2.1 cannot claim to predict the overall state of mental well-being in a country. First, it excludes information on mental health resources available in the general health system. But to that end, it does suggest a pattern, if perhaps a controversial one. Note that the services deemed necessary to a high-quality mental health system are located in ring-fenced facilities that are not integrated into the general health system. For example, countries with more psychiatric beds tend to house them in specialized psychiatric hospitals, not in the psychiatric wards of general hospitals (see WHO 2011, also Perera 2020a). Such ring-fencing may over-medicalize mental health (leaving less room for counseling and other less biomedically intensive social services) or make it difficult to integrate mental health care into the primary health system (an often lauded goal, see WHO 2014a).

Second, Figure 2.1 excludes the numerous other policy areas that support mental health. The person experiencing clinical depression, for example, may benefit from employment accommodations or disability insurance payments. The child with autism may benefit from specialized educational services. The person experiencing psychosis may require long-term housing assistance. Such "wrap-around" supports and structural factors matter greatly for overall psychological well-being (Allen et al. 2014; Johnson et al. 2015; WHO 2014b); however, the primary purpose of this book is to explain variations in the clinical services that address immediate mental health needs.

Put simply: To ensure *high-quality* mental health services, governments must first supply *services*. The noun is a prerequisite for its adjective. This data demonstrates that governments differ in the extent to which they succeed at that initial step. The varying supply presented in Figure 2.1 suggests that (1) some countries do provide mental health care at higher rates than expected by the "nowhere to go" narrative, (2) those high-supply countries tend to provide that care in both outpatient and hospital settings, and (3) mental health care supply depends heavily on public, not private, funding. The next section explores alternative explanations for these differences.

ALTERNATIVE EXPLANATIONS

To explain the puzzling differences in mental health care supply across countries, one might consider three alternative explanations. The first two, concerning the extent to which these differences align with cross-national differences in social welfare systems or health care systems, lose much of their explanatory power with a simple glance at Figure 2.1. The third, concerning the extent to which these differences result from varying historical differences in mental health care, requires a bit more unpacking. I will discuss that explanation in more depth after reviewing the first two, though it, too, is insufficient.

First, does a given country's "world of welfare" predict its mental health system? If Esping-Andersen's (1990) classic three-part typology of social welfare systems could explain mental health care systems, each country's placement in Figure 2.1 would be similar to that of others with similar social welfare systems. In other words, the "liberal" anglophone countries of Europe, North America, and Oceania, the "conservative" countries of continental Western Europe, and the "social democratic" countries of Nordic Europe would form distinct clusters on the graph. But this typological sorting is not visible in the figure. Although some of the smaller, more privatized welfare states of the liberal countries cluster at the lower end of the spectrum, others (Australia, England) supply mental health care at higher levels than the rest. Meanwhile, the generous social democratic welfare states, which typically supply public services at high levels, provide widely different amounts of mental health care (see the varying positions of Sweden, Denmark, Finland, and Norway). Continental European welfare states, whose attributes place them in between the liberal and social democratic extremes, furthermore, hardly follow any patterns at all.

Austria supplies mental health care at levels similar to both Canada and Sweden (a liberal and social democratic social welfare system). Yet some of Austria's continental siblings, Germany, Belgium, and the Netherlands, sit on the other end of the spectrum and off the line of best fit. As such, the factors that explain the variation in social welfare systems, in particular the political power afforded to the Left, would be unable to fully explain the variation in mental health care systems.

Second, does a given country's general health system predict its mental health care system? General health systems can vary in many ways, but one central dimension of variation is the relationship between providers (typically, physicians) and the government. Where providers have less autonomy, governments have more control and often oversee a fully public, state-owned health care system. Yet it is not clear that the supply of public mental health care is also greater in these countries. If that were the case, the supply of mental health care and the generosity of public financing would be universally high in countries with a national health service (i.e., Britain, Italy, and the Nordic countries), but it is not. It is curious that some countries with social insurance systems (e.g., Belgium, France, Germany) provide far more public mental health care than many of the national health service countries. But even within that subset of countries, there is significant variation in the quantity and distribution of mental health care services (e.g., low overall supply in Austria, higher-than-average community care in Germany, high inpatient care in Belgium). Since providers tend to have more bargaining power over the state in these countries, it is possible that those working in psychiatry may have greater institutional tools at their disposal to advocate for better pay and protections. But I will argue that the degree and scope of their success depends on other factors, namely their prospects for coalition with providers across occupational strata. As a result, what might explain the varying relationships between governments and providers across countries, such as the presence of institutional veto points, cannot wholly account for the variation in mental health care systems (Immergut 1992).

Other health system typologies fail to explain the variation in mental health care services as well (for a review, see Wendt and Bambra 2020). For example, countries with a high overall supply of general health care, public and private, do not necessarily have a high supply of mental health care as well. Neither do Reibling's (2010) "low supply" health care systems, such as Denmark, the Netherlands, and the United Kingdom, provide especially low levels of mental health care; nor does Moran's (2000) paradigmatic "supply state," the United States, provide especially high levels of it. Another example: Typologies that focus on the user experience in the general health system do not appear to account for that of the mentally ill. The "social democratic" health systems, for instance, reduce the extent to which patients must depend on the market for care (i.e., the extent to which the patient is "de-commodified," see Bambra 2005). Yet many of these countries, such as Canada, New Zealand, and Sweden, supply very low levels of public mental health care. The experiences of patients with mental illness, then, are different from those of others. In short, mental health care systems stand apart, producing politics, services, and experiences that do not resemble those in the general health system.

A third possible explanation considers the role of legacy: Does a given country's historical supply of mental health care predict its current supply of care in this area? Perhaps the countries with high levels of institutional care never deinstitutionalized in the first place. Or perhaps prior levels of inpatient care can explain contemporary levels. Assessing the validity of this genre of explanation requires both developing a clear, portable definition of deinstitutionalization and collecting the appropriate longitudinal and cross-national indicators. As the coda to this chapter describes, I define (psychiatric) deinstitutionalization as a society's movement down a continuum, in which the mentally ill become less likely to reside in an establishment that provides both psychiatric and custodial care than in the past. To measure this process across the full universe of cases (the 16 countries in Figure 2.1), editions of each country's national statistical yearbook were surveyed to obtain data from before, during, and after deinstitutionalization, from 1935 to about 2000 (see the Appendix for more information). Although not all indicators were available for all countries and all years, most of the yearbook editions consulted included some information on three of the most important indicators: the residential population, the number of mental hospitals, and the number of psychiatric beds.

To assess whether all countries deinstitutionalized, Figure 2.2 draws on an original data set (see the Appendix) to plot the primary indicator of this process: the proportion of residents in mental hospitals per 100,000 population in a given year, compared to the historical baseline (1935). It shows that all countries deinstitutionalized the resident population of mental hospitals, though the extent to which they did so varied substantially. In most cases, the likelihood of institutionalization in fact increased after the Second World War but began to decrease by the 1970s. An exception to this pattern is Switzerland, where institutionalization rates remained high in the 1970s and 1980s; and unfortunately no recent residential data is available for that country, so what happened after that period is unclear. The figure also suggests that historical levels of institutionalization cannot predict what occurred during deinstitutionalization itself. For example, countries that had some of the highest postwar rates of institutionalization, such as Canada and Australia, eventually came to have some of the lowest.[6]

To assess whether historic differences in inpatient care explain contemporary differences, Figures 2.3 and 2.4 plot observations from the original database on the supply of mental health care – hospitals and beds, respectively – in these countries.[7] They do not. While the supply of mental health care in countries like Austria, Australia, Sweden, and Canada was once above average, it is now well below it (compare to Figure 2.1). The opposite is true for countries such as France and Germany. In the case of Finland, institutional services even increased (even as the population residing in them decreased, see Figure 2.2). Also worth noting is that, prior to 1935, these countries governed public mental health services in very different ways. As Ansell and Lindvall (2020, table 7.1, 183) document, state control of asylums was common in Austria, Denmark, Finland, Germany, New Zealand, Norway, and Sweden; yet that control did not seem to stall the reduction of public institutional care in those countries with any consistency. In fact, contemporary levels of public mental health supply now vary widely.[8]

---

[6] It may come as a surprise that governments once supplied hospital services to indigent populations at high levels. But indigent "indoor relief" (e.g., asylums, orphanages, poor houses) was the standard form of welfare provision prior to the development of "outdoor relief" (e.g., cash assistance benefits and social insurance schemes) in the mid 20th century. Critical histories tend to explain these shifts by pointing to changing political-economic background conditions. The industrial transition of the late 19th century prompted governments to expand asylums to absorb unused surplus labor (Rothman 1971, 1980). Indoor relief was less necessary by the mid 20th century, as state formation processes facilitated the expansion of outdoor relief (Scull 1984).

[7] To simplify and summarize the trends, Figures 2.3 and 2.4 plot data from the earliest and latest available years and countries. Countries varied in whether and how they measured institutional care over time, so data on both hospitals and beds can provide a fuller picture of trends in institutional care. Note, too, how hospitals and beds do not necessarily correlate. Sweden, Canada, and Australia, for example, ranked highly on bed supply but low on hospital supply in 1935. Countries like those might provide many beds in a few large hospitals, while others provide fewer beds in many small hospitals. See also the coda to this chapter.

[8] Another important dimension of variation in public service governance for Ansell and Lindvall (2020, table 7.1, 183), the degree of centralization or decentralization, does not seem linked to contemporary levels of supply, either; the mechanism that might link these variables, furthermore, is not clear (as I will discuss in subsequent chapters).

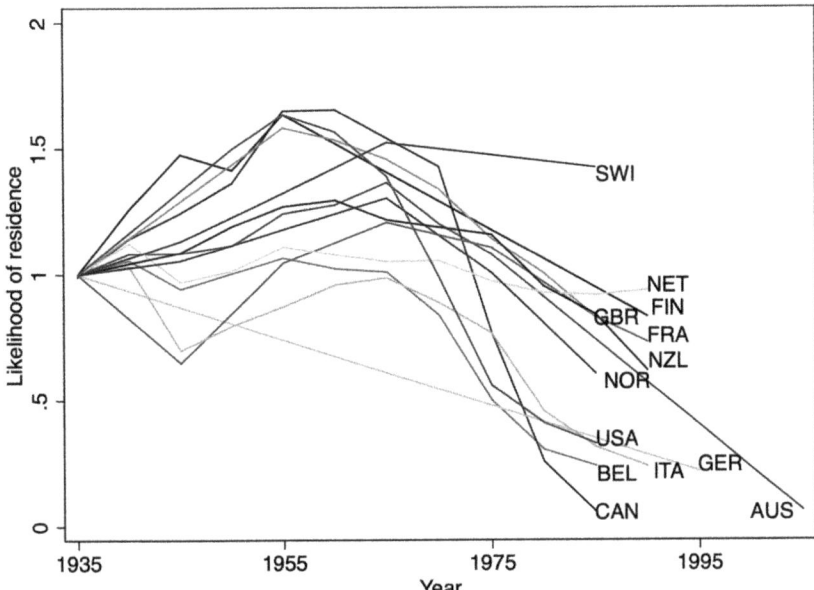

FIGURE 2.2 Residents of psychiatric hospitals per 100,000 people, relative to a 1935 baseline, available countries and years

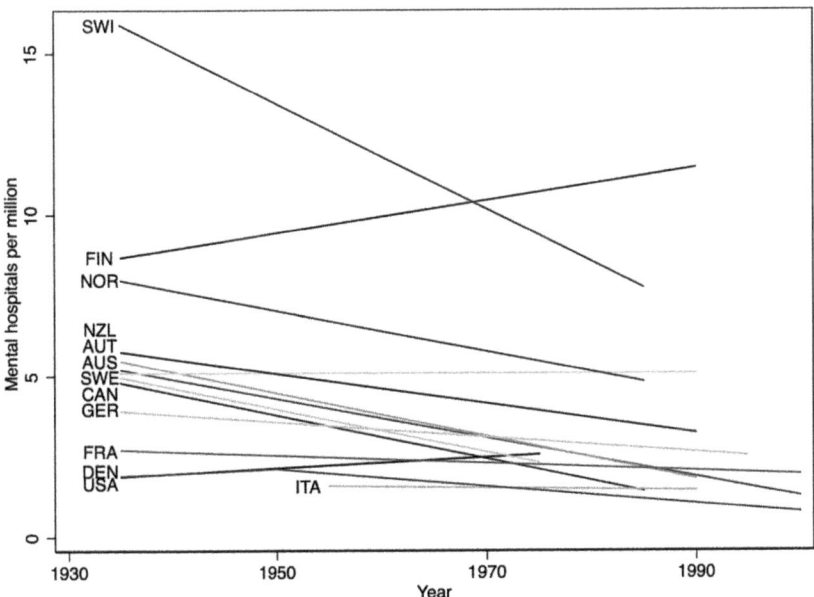

FIGURE 2.3 Mental hospitals per million people, 1935–2000, available countries and years

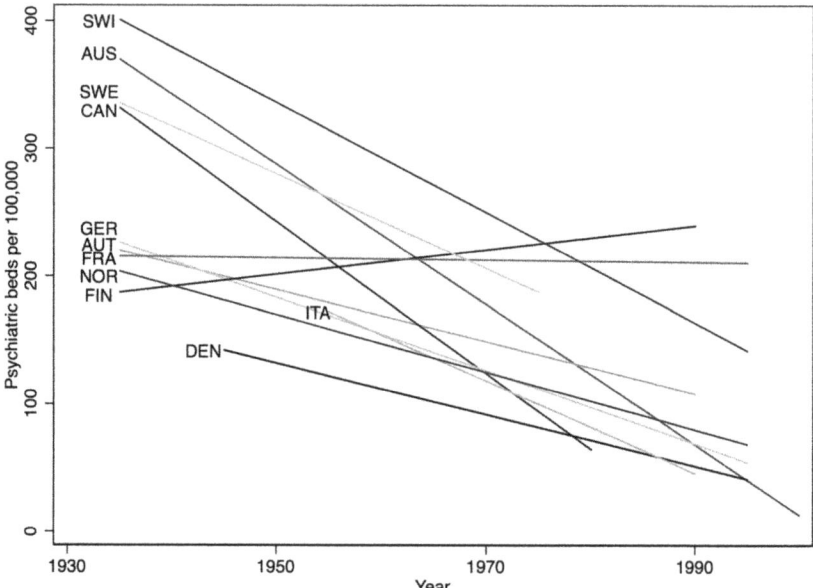

FIGURE 2.4 Psychiatric beds per 100,000 people, 1935–2000, available countries and years

Together, Figures 2.2–2.4 hence challenge the notion that countries with historically high levels of mental health care, especially institutional care, did not deinstitutionalize at the end of the 20th century. That all countries eventually deinstitutionalized makes theoretical sense, even if not all cases have been closely documented by historians and country experts. Following Scull's (1984) structural explanation for deinstitutionalization, in each of these countries favorable economic conditions in the postwar period expanded social insurance programs that would facilitate life outside the asylum, and the unfavorable economic conditions that followed in the 1970s and 1980s prompted governments to close costly inpatient mental health services. With the new antipsychotic medications, hospitals could reduce coercive restraint and outpatient treatment became more feasible. Developed by the French pharmaceutical company Rhône-Poulenc in the 1950s, chlorpromazine (also known under the trade names Thorazine and Largactil) was the first drug to treat psychosis (Grob 1991, 146–155; Scull 1984, 80). Although it was marketed, prescribed, and purchased in all these societies, chlorpromazine had little effect on the actual closure of hospitals (Gronfein 1985). In addition, the societal support for deinstitutionalization tended to be high in all western societies in the latter half of the

20th century. These movements, moreover, were transnational. Optimistic postwar reformers from more than 27 countries regularly met in Geneva to discuss their shared ambitions to transform mental health care (Henckes 2009; WHO 1978; see also Roelcke et al. 2010). Critics of institutional psychiatric power included Americans such as Erving Goffman, Alfred H. Stanton and Morris S. Schwartz, and Thomas Szasz; their counterparts in the British Commonwealth such as R. D. Laing and David Cooper; as well as non-anglophone thinkers such as Franco Basaglia and Frantz Fanon.[9] A steadily intensifying media spotlight on some of the most deplorable mental hospitals, accruing legal battles over involuntary commitment procedures, and the revolutionary overtones of the 1960s helped many of these ideas spread around the world. In sum, the three factors that helped to reduce the resident population of mental hospitals – movements, medications, and money – were present across each of these countries.

This data also challenges the notion that prior levels of institutionalization determined contemporary levels. The countries that provide greater levels of inpatient care today have not always done so. Notice also that, while most countries reduced the supply of psychiatric beds over the course of the 20th century, they did not necessarily do so by closing mental hospitals. Ironically, some countries reduced their resident population while increasing or generally maintaining the hospital and bed supply (Finland, France, Germany); Switzerland, meanwhile, saw dramatic supply reductions that do not match its residential trends in Figure 2.2. Since the varying supply of care today does not align with the variations prior to deinstitutionalization, then something must have occurred during deinstitutionalization to shift national policy trajectories. The next section presents a research strategy to explore those changes and test a hypothesis that can explain them.

RESEARCH DESIGN

As discussed in Chapter 1, this book proposes that the "welfare work-force" – the workers who depend on the welfare state for their employ-ment – shape social policy, particularly when its clients lack political power and as the underlying economic structure hangs on service industries

---

[9] Many would add the work of Michel Foucault (1961) to this list, though I refrain from doing so, as he attempted to distance himself somewhat from this group. Unlike the other thinkers, who critiqued contemporaneous institutions of psychiatric power, the French social theorist took a longer-term view on how capitalist development shaped the construction of madness itself. With the development of bourgeois values in the 17th century, he argued, madness became "incapacity for work," to which capitalist societies responded with a "great confinement."

such as health care and education. Psychiatric deinstitutionalization overlapped with this service transition, such that the increasing numbers of public mental health workers had the opportunity to influence policy in that area. But they were not always successful. Where they had access to political resources and allies, public sector workers were able to secure higher wages, more employment, and generous protections, a combination that results in more public services and feeds resources back into the workforce. This "supply-side policy feedback" process can be either positive or negative. Where workers did not have access to these supports, lower wages, fewer jobs, and layoffs resulted, producing fewer public services (see Figure 1.1, Chapter 1). To predict the likelihood of workers' success, I hypothesize that independently organized and unified public sector managers are more likely to advocate with their employees and, by extension, increase their political power. The presence of a "public labor–management coalition" – an especially potent alliance that is particular to the public sector – therefore can drive expansions in public services, even when beneficiaries (like the mentally ill) cannot demand them.

Testing the effect of this hypothesis on the development of a macro-level structural outcome such as mental health policy requires case analysis, since it allows paying full attention to the exploration of causes. Careful consideration of the "causes of effects" is a characteristic strength of case study research, for it unveils multilevel, evolving, and often unquantifiable causal factors and mechanisms (Mahoney and Terrie 2008). If this study is to unpack the political influence of public employees on mental health care, it must consider the shifting preferences of multiple actors (workers, managers, policy-makers) and their multiple representatives (trade unions, associations, government agencies) on various policy issues (inpatient care, outpatient care, public investment in psychiatric services). The same is true of historical developments (e.g., the growth of the public sector workforce, ideological change) and important cross-national differences (e.g., patterns of policy-making, demographic differences). Case studies make it possible to examine each of these complex factors in close detail and to assess their overall causal role more holistically.

Of the countries identified in Figure 2.1, two stand out as especially well-suited for detailed case comparison: the United States and France. The US experience of deinstitutionalization is, by far, the one that has most influenced popular and scholarly understandings of that process. If the proposed hypothesis found empirical support in this paradigmatic case, it would also call international presumptions about deinstitutionalization into question. In particular, evidence suggesting that the absence of a public labor–management coalition in the United States reduced the supply of all public mental health services in the late 20th century would challenge arguments about the functional, apolitical nature of deinstitutionalization, as well as about the necessity of closing hospitals to expand community care. France, by contrast, lies on the other extreme of the supply spectrum compared to the American case (see Gerring 2014). The expansive public mental health system in France developed during – even in spite of – psychiatric deinstitutionalization.

What renders this pairing most apt for comparison, though, is that a mid 20th-century observer could not have predicted these 21st-century policy outcomes (see Mahoney and Goertz 2004). If anything, the opposite might have been more likely. While the two countries shared a similar political economy of mental health care prior to deinstitutionalization and developed similar plans to reform it in the postwar period, policymakers in the United States initially benefited from better prospects for service expansion. The supply of public mental health care in France had suffered during the Second World War, while infrastructure was more robust in the United States. Moreover, commitment to the reform was stronger in the United States (where Congress enacted it into law) than in France (where an administrative circular merely suggested the idea).

But the possibility of coalition between public sector psychiatric managers and workers differed. In the 19th century, public sector psychiatric managers in both countries organized independently from those in the private sector, but by the early 20th century those in the United States opted to include private practitioners in their membership. This decision would set the United States on a very different pathway to deinstitutionalization after the Second World War. Chapter 3 hence uses the logic of the structured, paired comparison to both document these similar initial conditions and highlight a single difference of causal importance (Slater and Ziblatt 2013; Tarrow 2010).

Holding constant these otherwise similar initial conditions, US and French mental health policy diverged after the Second World War.[10]

---

[10] Figure 2.3 begins to document this divergence, though its degree may be difficult to perceive in the graph. In 1935, the supply of mental hospitals in both France and the United States ranked below the western average; but by 2000 that amount had reduced much more in the United States (by about 60 percent, or from 1.9 to 0.8 hospitals per million) compared to France (by just under 25 percent, or from 2.7 to 2.0 hospitals per million). When coupled with significant expansions to non-hospital mental health care (Figure 2.1 and documented in subsequent chapters), French mental health care supply ultimately exceeded that of the United States after deinstitutionalization.

Chapters 4 and 5 therefore separate the two cases, respectively, and use within-case process-tracing techniques to assess the validity of the proposed hypothesis against context-specific alternative explanations in each country. Chapter 4 explores whether the absence of independently organized and unified public sector managers in the United States foreclosed the possibility of coalition with their employees and facilitated negative supply-side policy feedback. Chapter 5 explores whether the coalition's presence in France enabled the opposite outcomes. Together, these two chapters examine whether and how a public labor–management coalition shaped policy feedback processes in mental health from the 1960s to the 1980s in these two main cases.

An abbreviated comparison of two other cases, Sweden and Norway, examines whether the argument can explain mental health care outcomes elsewhere. These two countries have much in common, such as their generous, state-oriented welfare states and large, powerful public sector workforces. Yet Sweden and Norway diverge widely on public mental health care. In fact, simply crossing the border from Norway into Sweden reduces the inpatient care supply by 60 percent. Community care is higher in Norway than Sweden as well. Support for the hypothesis in these two cases would bolster its predictive power. Analyses of Sweden and Norway can also refute alternative hypotheses that arise in the United States and France. For example, the role of the state is as important in Swedish welfare provision as it is in France (if not more so), yet Sweden did not produce the high levels of public mental health services accomplished by France. The decentralized Norwegian system, meanwhile, did not produce the rapid, "race to the bottom" deinstitutionalization experienced in the decentralized American welfare state. Chapter 6 presents the results of this second paired comparison.

Analyzing these four country cases has additional benefits. Together, they test the argument across all three types of welfare states (liberal America, conservative France, and social democratic Norway and Sweden) and across general health systems that are more oriented toward the private sector (France and the United States) compared to those oriented toward the public sector (Norway and Sweden). These cases also offer an opportunity to revise the standard narrative about better-known cases (the United States and, to some extent, Sweden) as well as to contribute to the English-language literature of lesser-known cases (France and Norway). Across all four cases, deinstitutionalization *did* occur (the population of patients residing in mental hospitals declined), but its outcomes differed. In the United States and Sweden, hospitals closed wholesale and few community services developed. By contrast, France and Norway kept existing hospital structures open while also expanding community services, in ways perhaps better aligned with the comprehensive goals of deinstitutionalization (see the coda to this chapter). The following section details these contemporary outcomes across the four cases.

OVERVIEW OF THE FOUR MENTAL HEALTH CARE
SYSTEMS SELECTED FOR COMPARISON

Countries That Supply Limited Public Mental Health Care Services

The United States

Since psychiatric deinstitutionalization, the supply of public mental health care has declined in the United States. During that time (1960s–1980s), the psychiatric bed capacity of state and county mental hospitals reduced by 70 percent and about one out of every five hospitals closed (Fisher et al. 2009). Although some policy-makers attempted to develop and expand a network of public community mental health centers (CMHCs), only a fraction of these 1,200 sites were built. Fewer have been maintained. Today, the vast majority of people requiring outpatient mental health care services must seek it in the private sector, often with hefty user fees (Druss et al. 2008). Out-of-pocket payments for US mental health services are quite high: about 11 percent of total spending (Garfield 2011). Some inpatient care is available at general hospitals, private psychiatric hospitals, military hospitals, and correctional facilities (SAMHSA 2010, tables 48 and 116). The latter is often a last resort that compensates for the lack of chronic psychiatric care capacity in the general health system.

As a result, access to mental health care is poor in the United States. Only about a third of Americans with mental health problems receive treatment (Cunningham 2009). Most outpatient visits are restricted to dispensing medication, not therapeutic or rehabilitative services (Olfson and Marcus 2010). Moreover, the limitations of public mental health care and financing mean that private psychiatry is not only dominant in the United States but also its accessibility is limited to the most affluent of patients; those who can afford to pay the full cost of these services. Less affluent Americans are more likely to find themselves in prisons or homeless shelters than in psychiatric hospitals or clinics; psychiatric conditions affect about half of incarcerated individuals and about a quarter of chronically homeless individuals (Culhane 2008; James and Glaze 2006). In effect, this group has "nowhere (else) to go."[11]

Contemporary public policies structure these supply and access outcomes. Public mental hospitals, originally financed by state and county mental hospitals, began to close when the federal Social Security program developed in the 1960s and 1970s. Several new social programs incentivized states to shift patients to non-hospital settings. Medicaid, a joint state–federal public insurance program for the poor and disabled enacted in 1965, refused to pay for services in "institutions for mental disease" (IMDs, or specialized adult psychiatric institutions with more than 16 beds; hereafter the "IMD Exclusion"); however Medicaid would pay for long-term care services for the elderly, who composed a significant portion of the institutionalized population at the time.[12] Those payments, combined with a congressional support for nursing home construction, shifted much of the patient population from state and county mental hospitals to nursing homes. Meanwhile, Social Security Insurance, the disability insurance program enacted in 1972, also discouraged public inpatient psychiatry by denying benefits to individuals living in public institutions, such as state and county mental hospitals. Finally, Medicare, the income-taxed public insurance program for the aged and the disabled, would cover only 190 days of inpatient psychiatric care (in any institution, public or private) over the beneficiary's lifetime. These changes have weakened the financial support for inpatient mental health care over time.

Community mental health care faced similar policy constraints. Congress enacted the CMHC program for only a few years at a time, limited the funds available for staff, and eventually structured it as a block-grant program. These factors stalled its expansion. Private insurers, which cover about two-thirds of the population, mostly through employment contributions, were not incentivized to cover outpatient care (or inpatient care); so they reimburse providers at low rates.[13] The same is

---

[11] Other countries with limited public mental health care face similar challenges, if not to the same extreme as the United States (see Willison and Mauri 2021).

[12] For in-depth reviews of the IMD Exclusion and its (limited) exceptions, see Houston 2023; Mitchell 2015; Zur et al. 2017.

[13] Not until the passage of the Affordable Care Act in 2010 were private health insurers demanded to cover a minimum basket of health benefits. Prior to the Act, moreover, private insurers were permitted to deny coverage on the basis of a preexisting health condition, such as a mental illness. The law now requires some new health plans to cover mental health services at "parity" (at the same rate as other specialty

true for both Medicare and Medicaid. According to Bishop et al. (2014), and as a consequence, only half of psychiatrists accept Medicare and private insurance and only 43 percent accept Medicaid, compared to nearly all physicians in other specialties (86, 89, and 73 percent, respectively). Thus, Chapter 4 will trace the political factors that produced these policy constraints in the United States.

Sweden

Sweden also has a limited supply of mental health care. Although mental health care provision is formally public and universal, public rhetoric has labeled it a "policy failure" and "national disgrace" (see the infamous comments of Social Democrat Lars Engqvist discussed in Chapter 6).[14] The poor reputation of Swedish mental health care is partly because it is not financially differentiated from general health care. There is no stand-alone fund for mental health care, since it depends on and competes for the same national funds that finance the general health system. As in the general health care system, 80 percent of mental health spending is funded by the national government and through public grants, while out-of-pocket payments account for 17 percent of expenditures (the remaining 4 percent is funded by marginal county and municipal taxes). Mental health care patients pay similar user fees as somatic patients, capped at just over $100 (USD) per year (NOMESCO-NOSOSCO 2022; per Riksbank 2022). Private psychiatric practitioners account for about 7 percent of total mental health care provision in Sweden (Anell et al. 2012; Glenngård 2020).

Another factor contributes to the low supply of mental health care in Sweden. As I will discuss in Chapter 6, in the 1990s the government devolved the responsibility for the nonmedical social care of the mentally ill to the municipal level. This move severed incentives for the regions to integrate medical and social – especially residential – services and resulted in significant cost-shifting to municipalities. Only very few dedicated funds are available to compensate them. Here, too, services depend on and compete for the same national funds (and marginal local taxes) for solvency. Significant local discretion in their allocation, moreover,

health care services); however, (1) plans may vary the scope of benefits they cover and (2) the regulations concerning this provision are difficult to implement at the state level, as previous legislative attempts have shown (see Dixon 2009; Frank et al. 1997; Garfield et al. 2010; Jensen et al. 1998; Manderscheid 2009; Rice et al. 2013; SAMHSA 2012).

[14] Lars Engqvist, interview, *Aktuellt*, Sveriges Television, January 3, 2000.

means that services for the mentally ill are often short-changed and vary by municipality, as noted in that chapter.

Countries That Supply Extensive Public Mental Health Care Services

France

Unlike the mental health systems just described, France expanded its mental health care system during psychiatric deinstitutionalization. The 1960s to 1980s saw the development of psychiatric "sectorization" instead. The sectors partition the country into more than 1,200 geographic catchment areas for populations of around 60,000–70,000 people. Each must provide multidisciplinary mental health care, though the precise mix of services depends on the perceived needs of the population.[15] Nonetheless, sectors include a public psychiatric outpatient care center (*centre médico-psychologique*) that offers ambulatory mental health care, coordinated by a public hospital (Chevreul et al. 2015). Care is available outside of the sectorization system as well. Although public sectorized services are more diverse and more numerous than private mental health services, the private sector accounts for about 20 percent of inpatient cases and about 50 percent of outpatient psychiatrists (Chevreul et al. 2010; DREES 2016). Moreover, sectors are supplemented by a range of "medical-social" services (*services médico-sociaux*), such as housing, educational support, professional training, and sheltered workshops. The degree of coordination between the sectors and these public or not-for-profit medical-social services varies. This is partly because of the differences in their client populations, the psychiatric sectors care for more people with mental disabilities than medical-social services do (Chevreul et al. 2015, table 5.3), and partly because of the competition between them. As a result, sectorization has remained, in the words of one influential government report, the "basic organizing principle" of psychiatry in France (Piel and Roelandt 2001).

Sectorization helps to promote high levels of access to mental health care in France, where the utilization of psychiatric services is higher than in many of its peer societies, including Great Britain and Denmark (DGC 2014). But even within France, mental health care is considered more accessible than other forms of health care. The major government

---

[15] The term "multidisciplinary" refers to the care provided by a variety of practitioners, including psychiatrists, psychiatric nurses, psychologists, and social workers.

agency for health statistics (the *Direction de la recherche, des études, de l'évaluation et des statistiques*, or DREES) rates access to psychiatrists higher than access to pediatricians. In urban areas, psychiatrists are more accessible than ophthalmologists and gynecologists (Castell and Dennevault 2017).

These supply and access outcomes, too, are the product of public policy. As Chapter 5 will show, the sectorization system grew out of a small community care program that eventually gained long-term financial support from the general health system. Today, French health insurance funds (financed by employment contributions and other revenues) entitle all residents to a basket of preapproved health care services, including psychiatric services (Mossialos et al. 2017). In general, services rendered at public institutions require an up-front payment of 20 euro, while private providers require more (at least 25 euro), but this difference is much wider in mental health care services: 15 euro for public providers and at least 39.70 euro for private providers. The funds then reimburse 70 percent of public sector fees and 30 percent of the negotiated private sector fees, but beneficiaries with chronic conditions such as mental illness qualify for full reimbursement of these fees. In short, these financial arrangements cover virtually all health costs for people with mental illness and incentivize the development of public psychiatric care.

Norway

Norway also provides high levels of mental health care. To understand why, it is crucial to understand its distinct financial and administrative infrastructure. The state often provides a substantial pot of separate public funding for mental health. A "Golden Rule" principle even stipulates that growth in mental health care must be greater than growth in general somatic health care (Romøren 2018).[16] Norway has also implemented a system similar to French "sectorization." Drawing on centralized general tax revenues, municipalities administer and pay for "district psychiatric centers," public psychiatric outpatient care centers akin to the *centres médico-psychologiques*. They also pay for, manage, and integrate these services into the municipalities' inpatient psychiatry. Regional health authorities pay other outpatient care (about half of the total supplied). These patterns produce some geographic variation

---

[16] In contrast to mental health care, somatic health care addresses a patient's physical needs.

in service supply; but unlike their counterparts in Sweden (or even the United States), Norwegian localities draw on far fewer local funds to provide care. Instead, they rely equally on funds distributed from the central government and must commit to providing a basic package of services in exchange for it. Although the vast majority of care is public, 12 percent is provided through private practitioners contracted by specialty hospitals (Sperre Suanes 2020). Moreover, children receiving care in the district psychiatric centers and their attendant hospitals have no payment. The same is true for adults who have reached the yearly user fee ceiling limit (about $240 USD, NOMESCO-NOSOSCO 2022; per Norges Bank 2023a).

The examples of France and Norway challenge the narrative that people with mental conditions have "nowhere to go" for care. Although that might be true in the United States and the other countries on the low end of the spectrum plotted in Figure 2.1, it is not true for all affluent democracies. In fact, and contrary to scholarly and popular presumptions of mental health, countries that supply high levels of mental health care provide both ample community care and ample inpatient care through the public sector. As noted, existing typologies of national public policy approaches cannot explain these differences. Moreover, the variation exists despite countries' shared experience of psychiatric deinstitutionalization.

A comparative-historical analysis can test the hypothesis that the presence of a public labor–management coalition, enabled by independently organized and unified public managers, propelled the welfare workforce to expand mental health care in some countries (while absence of the welfare workforce reduced mental health care in others). Four cases, whose contemporary mental health systems have been discussed in this chapter, will serve as the testing ground for this hypothesis in the chapters that follow. Chapters 3–5 first assesses the hypothesis in the case of US deinstitutionalization, which most influenced global narratives about this process, against the contrasting experience in France. Chapter 3 structures the comparison by ensuring that the conditions that preceded deinstitutionalization were the same in both countries, save for the organization of their public psychiatric managers. Chapters 4 and 5 use within-case process-tracing techniques to show how this difference shaped the diverging trajectories of deinstitutionalization in the United States and France, respectively. Chapter 6 then assesses the extent to which the hypothesis can explain the supply of mental health care elsewhere (and account for lingering alternative hypotheses) by juxtaposing the cases of Sweden and

Norway. Together, I leverage these four cases to demonstrate how the welfare workforce shaped the supply of mental health care across a variety of welfare state regimes, health system types, and time periods.

CODA: DEINSTITUTIONALIZATION DEFINED

Conceptualizing deinstitutionalization requires determining whether to use that term in the first place. In humanistic and social science theory, institutionalization most often refers to the normalizing, routinizing, or codifying of various aspects of social life. Meanwhile, in the empirical analysis of social policy, the term can apply to multiple areas, such as the historic deinstitutionalization of workers out of poorhouses, or of children out of orphanages, and even the institutionalization of the elderly into care homes.[17]

Even among scholars of mental health, the term lacks universal acceptance. Critical scholars concerned with the evolution of social control techniques have opted for language with a stronger charge. The influential writings of Andrew Scull (1984, 1), for example, employ the term "decarceration" to refer to a broader "state-sponsored policy of closing down asylums, prisons, and reformatories." At the same time, scholars writing about non-anglophone countries often find that this anti-institutional bias does not represent the experiences of other countries. Writing about the French experience, Henckes (2009, 511–18) "questions the deinstitutionalization model as an explanation of transformations of the structure of the French psychiatry system in the postwar period," noting that not all societies "call[ed] into question the psychiatric hospitals themselves."

Nevertheless, the term "deinstitutionalization" remains the language of choice for many academics and journalists commenting on the psychiatric

---

[17] In fact, deinstitutionalization is vital to welfare state formation. Consider Karl Polanyi's classic 1944 analysis of the Speenhamland system in early industrial England. The Great Transformation reveals how shifting welfare provision from the institutional ("indoor relief") to the noninstitutional ("outdoor relief") eventually resulted in the dual protection and regulation of labor for capitalist development. Similar trends would take off in North America, where students of US social history would come to emphasize the role of both institutionalization (e.g., Rothman 1971) and deinstitutionalization (e.g., Katz 1996) in welfare capitalism. Over the coming decades, deinstitutionalization would take many forms. Lerman (1982) identifies three types of deinstitutionalization in 20th-century America alone: the deinstitutionalization of the mentally ill from state hospitals, that of the developmentally disabled from specialized state schools, and that of neglected and deviant youth from orphan asylums and training schools.

experience (e.g., Goodwin 1997; Harcourt 2011; Mechanic and Rochefort 1990; Scheff 2014; Pan 2013; Ford 2015). Thus, while it is necessary to acknowledge the aforementioned limitations of the term, my focus on mental health policy prompts me to use this familiar and resonant language – two important criteria for concept formation (Gerring 1999).

Most analysts share an understanding that deinstitutionalization involves a shift in the primary locus of mental health services from one type of institution (namely, a mental hospital or asylum) to the community. What they mean by a "shift" and "community," however, varies. The shift can involve either the reduction of the number of institutional residents or a reduction in the number of institutions themselves. Although I use the contemporary WHO definition of community-based care, the meaning of this term has evolved over time. When deinstitutionalization began to acquire political significance in the 1970s and 1980s, scholars began pointing to an increased reliance on "nontraditional" or "noninstitutional" mental health care facilities (Bachrach 1983). Today, these facilities range from outpatient psychiatric centers, to nonmedical social services such as day care and vocational rehabilitation services, and even to housing facilities such as group homes and halfway houses. The varied meanings and usages of the term "deinstitutionalization" fail to provide a portable standard for comparison across countries.

Goertz's (2020) guidelines for concept formation can help to remedy this problem. At a "basic" level, degrees of institutionalization refer to whether the mentally ill in a given society are more or less likely to reside in an establishment that provides both psychiatric and custodial care. Deinstitutionalization, therefore, refers to a society's movement down a continuum, in which the mentally ill become less likely to reside in these establishments than in the past. Three components of this definition, and the indicators used to measure them, warrant highlighting and discussion in greater detail: the psychiatric-custodial establishment, the length of residence, and the relative likelihood of residence. Table 2.1 offers a schematic guide to this overview.

The presence or absence of the *psychiatric-custodial establishment* is perhaps the most visible marker of institutionalization. The decoupling of psychiatric and custodial care developed over the latter half of the 20th century, making these establishments appear obsolete to contemporary observers. While many specialized psychiatric hospitals still provide medical care, rarely do they serve a custodial function as well. Importantly, this dimension assumes that the society in question has a tradition of caring for the mentally ill in asylums. The repurposing or

TABLE 2.1 *Schematic of the concept and measurement of "deinstitutionalization"*

Basic definition	A society's movement down a continuum, in which the mentally ill become less likely to reside in an establishment that provides both psychiatric and custodial care than in the past		
Dimensions	Prevalence of establishments that provide both psychiatric services and custodial care	The degree of permanence with which people with mental illness are institutionalized	Relative likelihood of residence in these establishments
Indicator example	Number of mental hospitals	Length of stay in mental hospitals	Proportion of residents in mental hospitals per 100,000 population in a given year, compared to a historical baseline (e.g., 1935)

decline of the asylum constitutes this critical dimension of deinstitutionalization. To measure this dimension, the most obvious indicator is the number of establishments themselves; but looking only at the availability of mental hospitals says little about whether they serve a custodial function, in addition to a medical function. Substitute indicators, such as utilization rates (e.g., admissions) and capacity (e.g., beds) present the same problem, perhaps even more so, since these measures sometimes reflect the activity of both mental hospitals and the psychiatric wards of general hospitals.

Since these indicators do not convey very much information about how mental health care has changed within the hospital, the *length of residence* dimension attempts to capture changes in the function of the hospital, specifically regarding its custodial work. This component refers to the degree of permanence with which people with mental illnesses are institutionalized. Substitutable, constitutive indicators of this dimension include the average length of stay in a psychiatric institution and measures of long-term residents (sometimes called "inmates"). Note that inpatients can be distinct from residents. Inpatients can include those who stay in a mental hospital temporarily (even just one or two days), while residence connotes a long-term care arrangement.

Finally, the dimension of *relative likelihood* ties it all together. It shows that long-stay residence in the psychiatric-custodial establishment is changing over time. It captures, first, the likelihood that a person with mental illness resides in a mental hospital and, second, whether that person is any more or less likely to reside there today than in the past. It hence compares two populations (the institutionalized mentally ill to the noninstitutionalized mentally ill) and two time periods (the likelihood of institutionalization in one period in time to its likelihood in a previous period). Indicators of the effect of this phenomenon must capture the proportion of the population at a point in time that could be institutionalized, relative to a historical baseline. An ideal indicator is the percentage of residents living in mental hospitals, relative to those living in mental hospitals in 1935, well in advance of deinstitutionalization and just before the Second World War began. Setting the baseline during the war itself would have to account for war-induced population changes, particularly in the countries where the war was fought. The year 1935 offers a slightly more standardized baseline.

Measures of deinstitutionalization should consider the psychiatric needs of the population, too; but it is possible to presume that needs have been and continue to be similar across countries Moreover, epidemiologists have difficulty estimating these needs, in part because they are often partially (sometimes entirely) constructed, as sociologists have long emphasized (Durkheim 1897; Parsons 1951; Scheff 1966). The evolving classification of psychiatric disorders make this patently clear (Bayer 1987; Grob 1991; Kirk and Kutchins 1992; Mayes and Horwitz 2005). Yet most western societies have used and continue to use broadly similar diagnostic categories. For this reason, it is likely that social perceptions of psychiatric needs were parallel across countries at any given point in time. For example, the perceived mental health needs in France in 1950 were comparable to the perceived mental health needs in Belgium in 1950. Major international observers agree implicitly. As previously mentioned, the WHO has found that neuropsychiatric conditions account for about 30 percent of the global burden of disease in every western society, even though the provision of services for these conditions varies across those countries (WHO 2011).

3

Before Deinstitutionalization

The United States and France Compared

The central empirical task of this book is to demonstrate that, all other things being about equal, alliances between the managers and employees of public mental health services shaped the trajectory of public policy in that area. That the United States and France meet this *ceteris paribus* condition might surprise some readers, who otherwise might view those two countries as far more different than the Scandinavian societies of Sweden and Norway. Moreover, the contemporary US and French mental health care systems appear to align with the general patterns of social provision in each country: limited and privatized on the one hand and generous and state-centric on the other. Yet these outcomes were less obvious prior to psychiatric deinstitutionalization in the second half of the 20th century. In fact, a midcentury observer might not have predicted that the supply of mental health in France would exceed that of the United States (see Figure 1.1 in Chapter 1). If anything, the opposite prediction could have been deemed more likely.

This chapter shows that the political-economic conditions that preceded French and US deinstitutionalization were broadly similar. At the close of the Second World War, both countries structured their social welfare and mental health care systems in comparable ways. They each began to experience the transformative period of economic growth and welfare expansion that rendered deinstitutionalization possible, and each approached that "Golden Age" with nearly identical blueprints for mental health reform. Of the two, though, the United States appeared to have the upper hand. The war had devastated mental health care provision in France: More than 40,000 patients had died of famine and dozens of hospitals had been bombed, closed, or otherwise requisitioned for military purposes. Meanwhile, the supply of services in the United States remained in regular use and offered a more robust infrastructure for future expansion, to which legislators had explicitly committed.

One difference, though, stands out between the two countries: the possibility of coalition formation between workers and managers in public mental health services. On the labor side, French public sector trade unions acquired full legal rights after the war, but the maturation of their US counterparts was late, limited, and staggered across the states. As a result, French public employees gained their political-economic voice precisely at a turning point of welfare state formation, while American workers were absent from parallel discussions in the United States. The present study emphasizes the effects of this difference on mental health policy; but worth noting is that the same difference likely impacted other policy areas as well. Indeed, the postwar welfare workforce may have shaped the general patterns of social provision in each country in ways not yet fully appreciated.

On the management side, French public psychiatric managers were better equipped to enter into this coalition than their American counterparts. A series of conflicts in the 19th and early 20th centuries had led public psychiatric managers to organize independently of private practitioners in France: They formed the Trade Union of Psychiatric Hospital Physicians (Syndicat des médecins des hôpitaux psychiatriques, hereafter simply referred to as the Syndicat). The same conflicts were present in the United States, but actors settled them differently. Over time, a single representative organization for both public and private practitioners emerged: the American Psychiatric Association. These institutional changes command significant attention in this chapter, since the different organizational outcomes may have been related to structural factors in the political economy of mental health in each country. The existing historical accounts, though, attribute those outcomes to specific intra-professional conflicts.

My analytic emphasis nonetheless departs from the standard historiography with an alternative account of intra-professional conflict. Behind the animosity between hospital superintendents (originally called "alienists"), neurologists, office-based practitioners, and academic researchers, I find there were significant economic cleavages as well. While the interests of hospital superintendents were tied closely to their public employment and role as administrators, those of the other, non-state, actors often favored private provision. These differences may not have appeared to be the center of the controversy at the time, but as the following pages will reveal, they were fundamental to how different types of psychiatrists perceived themselves and their interests. Similar cleavages were present in both cases, and for similar reasons, yet their settlements were negotiated and adapted in different ways in France and in the United States. As such, this analysis reveals the importance of political representation to the overall development of the psychiatric identity in each country, which in France became more aligned with public administration than in the United States.

By the end of the Second World War, similar conditions framed mental health care in the United States and France. One exception was that French public psychiatric managers had developed a unified and independent political voice they could ally with that of the newly legalized public sector trade unions. In contrast, American public sector managers had lost this unified and independent voice, and they also lacked a unionized coalition partner. These empirical differences hence lend evidence in support of the hypothesis articulated in Chapter 1: Provided the presence of labor rights, public labor–management coalitions are more likely to form when the organization of public managers is unified and independent of their private sector counterparts. Evidence for this chapter is drawn from secondary accounts of trade union and psychiatric history, authored primarily by area experts. Since few scholars have focused on the economic conflicts underpinning psychiatric history, however, primary sources also play an important role in the section on managerial organization. I have reviewed the academic journals and trade press of public and private psychiatric practitioners from the mid 1800s to just after the Second World War, in order to reinterpret key position statements and organizational rule-changes from an economic perspective. In France, these journals include the *Annales médico-psychologiques* (published from 1843 to the present), the *Rapports du Congrès des médecins aliénistes et neurologistes de France et des pays de langue française* (published from 1891 to 1957), and *l'Information psychiatrique* (published from 1945 to the present). In the United States, these journals include the *American Journal of Insanity* (1844–1920) and the *American Journal of Psychiatry* (1921 to the present). The chapter ends by reviewing potential confounding explanations, concluding that none offers a more convincing explanation for the eventual variation in mental health service provision across the two countries than the central hypothesis tested in this and subsequent chapters.

SIMILAR INITIAL CONDITIONS

For scholars of western welfare states, the Second World War was a critical historical juncture for social policy change. The same applies to mental health policy and the onset of psychiatric deinstitutionalization.

TABLE 3.1 *Similar initial conditions in postwar America and France (before psychiatric deinstitutionalization)*

	United States	France
Postwar economic growth and welfare expansion	"Golden Age"; Great Society	*Trente Glorieuses*; Laroque Report
Structure of social welfare provision, in general	Not universalized, occupation-based, dependent on local governments	
Structure of mental health care provision, specifically	Decentralized public administration of asylums	
Pressures to deinstitutionalize and blueprint for reform	Community mental health centers	Sectorization

A dramatic upheaval of international and domestic orders, the war (and its settlement) made new political opportunities possible (Capoccia and Kelemen 2007). The time was ripe for actors to make fresh public policies that would impact social life for decades to come. Efforts to reform mental health care, in particular, encountered similar political, economic, and social conditions in the French and American contexts. In fact, although public mental health care in France would eventually exceed that of the United States, these outcomes were hardly foregone conclusions in the early postwar period. Rather, the conditions listed in Table 3.1 rendered similar outcomes just as possible (Mahoney and Goertz 2004).

In both the United States and France, the postwar period was one of significant economic and welfare state expansion, conditions that Scull (1984) found launched the initial decline of mental hospital residents by facilitating their access to income, health, and social care outside the asylum's walls. The unprecedented prosperity of the French *Trente Glorieuses*, or the "thirty glorious years" between 1945 and 1975, produced high productivity, high average wages, and high consumption. Inspired in part by the 1942 British Beveridge Report, the 1962 Laroque Report subsequently launched the expansion and development of France's social benefit system. Parallel developments occurred in the United States. The economic growth of America's "Golden Age" opened the door to numerous social policy reforms, including the landmark "Great Society" expansions of the 1960s. In short, the basic political and economic conditions of the two postwar countries laid the necessary foundation for deinstitutionalization.

Not only was deinstitutionalization probable but several factors suggest that the process could have taken a similar character in the two countries. At the time, American and French social welfare policy operated according to a similar logic. Postwar health and social insurance schemes protected specific occupational groups, namely industrial, agricultural, commercial, and government workers. Although the two countries structured these schemes differently (with varied dependence on commercial insurance providers), their demographic impacts on public mental health care were comparable. Such coverage reduced the dependence of those occupational groups and, crucially, those retired from them, on mental hospitals. By the mid 20th century, mental hospitals in both countries (and elsewhere) also served as care homes for the elderly. Increased access to pension and health insurance schemes would facilitate the transition of older patients out of asylums and often into the burgeoning long-term care industry (Derrien and Rossigneux-Méheust 2020; Grob and Goldman 2006). Neither country, however, had universalized these benefits. As a result, care for the poor and destitute, the primary population of the mental hospital, depended on residual forms of welfare, which was largely under the purview of local governments.

As such, in both countries, subnational authorities – states in America, *départements* in France – managed a system of mostly public mental hospitals. From a legal perspective, the French system appeared more centralized than the American one. The American Constitution's Tenth Amendment left issues of health under the jurisdiction of state governments, while an 1838 French law required every *département* to supply an "asylum" (*Loi sur les aliénés du 30 juin 1838*). But French departmental councils, a local assembly of elected officials, set their own asylum budgets. While the central government provided the funds for these budgets (in contrast with the US approach), local authorities held significant control over the scale and distribution of care. As a result, budgets across *départements* could vary up to threefold (Chapireau 2022). Note also that the 1838 law did not finance asylum construction. As a result, *départements* constructed new public asylums in fits and starts, and only when economic conditions were propitious (Longin 1999). Moreover, many *départements* initially left this responsibility to the Church, a non-state actor (Goldstein 1987). Although public asylums gradually replaced religious institutions, the fact remains that France also relied on non-state mental health care.[1] This is

---

[1] Ben Ansell and Johannes Lindvall, "Mental Asylum History ≈ 1800–1939, England, France, Sweden, USA, Australia, Japan, Germany, Spain, Canada, Netherlands, Denmark, Norway, Ireland, Belgium, Austria, Switzerland, Italy, Finland and New Zealand." Unpublished draft text (accessed May 1, 2017).

perhaps another factor that could have biased France against the expansion of public mental health care after the Second World War.

The entwining issues of race and federalism could have posed additional constraints on the expansion of American public mental health care – though at the end of the Second World War, their possible effects were unclear. As scholars such as Robert Lieberman (1998) and Jill Quadagno (1994) have shown, powerful white Southern Democrats interested in maintaining a race-based and labor-repressive agricultural economy ensured that redistributive policy would not overturn that system, in part by reinforcing the tradition of local control. Ironically, however, the supply of mental health care in Southern states was often higher than elsewhere in the country (SAMHSA 1992, 50–51). Jim Crow-era laws concerning segregation produced separate, if highly unequal, facilities for Black patients (Edwards-Grossi 2021, 87). How the presence of these extra public facilities would affect the prospects for deinstitutionalization hence was unclear, especially since the carceral system had not yet begun to expand. As Anne Parsons (2018) has argued, not only did deinstitutionalization precede mass incarceration but deinstitutionalization was not the singular cause of mass incarceration, despite long-standing, simplified theories to the contrary (e.g., Penrose 1939).[2]

Both countries also shared a long tradition of private medical practice. In general, private providers delivered nonpsychiatric care. Reinforcing that pattern were the two countries' powerful medical professions. Codified in the statutes and founding documents of the main medical associations, the American Medical Association (AMA) and the Confederation of French Medical Trade Unions (Confédération des syndicats médicaux français, or CSMF), were firm commitments to direct price-setting between doctors and patients, fee-for-service payment, and market-based medical care (Dutton 2008). In both cases, therefore, the

---

[2] Less attention has been paid to the relationship between racialized political geography and welfare provision in France; so here, too, it is difficult to develop clear hypotheses about its effect on mental health care. France's overseas departments, most notably Algeria, may have shaped the distribution of metropolitan welfare in ways not yet fully explored in existing scholarship (though see Lyons 2013). The limited incorporation of Algerian Muslims into political institutions, for example, may have contributed to France's own fragmented, privatized approach to welfare at the time. Moreover, the war in Algeria (1954–62) and Algeria's subsequent independence triggered the formation of a more centralized Fifth Republic (Shepard 2008), which suggests that Algeria's presence in the French polity prior to that point may have played a similar role to that of the American South in the United States. As Lieberman's (2003) comparative work has explored, the very structure of French social policy may be related to the structure of the colonialist polity.

private sector preferences of the general medical profession could contest the public expansion of the mental health care system.

Perhaps the most notable commonality between postwar French and American mental health policy is that leaders in the two countries intentionally borrowed ideas from one another. Although the academic and social movement to deinstitutionalize the mentally ill would not gain prominence until the late 1960s and 1970s, by the 1950s the World Health Organization (WHO) was promoting global mental health reform among policy elites. In addition to convening regular meetings of its Expert Committee on Mental Health (over half of whose members were either French or American), the WHO also provided funds for participants to visit the psychiatric hospitals and clinics of other countries (Henckes 2009). When psychiatrist Maurice Despinoy returned to France from his WHO-sponsored American tour, for example, he brought with him the concept of the "day hospital" (Henckes 2007), an idea that later became integral to the expansive French public mental health care system, if not the more limited American one.

These meetings also contributed to the two countries' shared blueprint for reform. Geographically defined catchment areas – of about 60,000–70,000 people in France and between 75,000 and 200,000 people in the United States (Coldefy 2007, 23; Foley 1975, 92) – would provide a range of outpatient services for patients formerly cared for in mental hospitals. Hospitals, though, would continue to play an important role. Members of the Expert Committee, for example, viewed the average number of psychiatric hospital beds in western countries – about 3 per 1,000 inhabitants – as the new norm (Henckes 2009). Outpatient programs would supplement, not wholly replace, that inpatient care.

Closing the hospitals was by no means off the table. Although psychiatrists had begun to rethink its role, the institution remained an important part of psychotherapeutic treatment. Both "institutional psychotherapy" in France and "milieu therapy" (and to some extent "psychodynamics") in the United States viewed the hospital environment and its social life as an active form of treatment (Grob 1994, 226; Robcis 2021). Moreover, even the budding critiques of the asylum did not conclude that hospital care was destined for failure. For example, Albert Deutsch's proposed policy solution in his 1948 *The Shame of the States* called not for an end to the asylum but rather for additional public funding to hospitals to address the "twin diseases" of overcrowding and understaffing.[3]

---

[3] Note that the most influential public advocacy efforts tended to come from journalists like Deutsch, rather than the patients themselves. During the asylum period, especially,

Deutsch's policy prescriptions call attention to two factors that gave the United States an upper hand in implementing the above vision of reform. First, the overcrowding of postwar American hospitals stands in sharp contrast to the opposite development in French hospitals. Between 40,000 and 45,000 patients in French psychiatric hospitals had died of famine and neglect during the war (von Bueltzingsloewen 2007). Such devastation significantly reduced the utilization and contemporary relevance of psychiatric hospitals. Table 3.2 uses data from the previous chapter to compare patterns of hospital residency and supply in the two countries before and after deinstitutionalization.[4] Note how the population-adjusted rate of institutional residency in France is nearly 30 percent less than that of the United States in 1955, and how that relationship flips dramatically in 1985. Moreover, although the supply of hospitals is somewhat lower in the United States compared to France in 1955, it drops even further over the course of deinstitutionalization while the French levels remain the same.

These diverging outcomes are surprising for a second reason: American policy-makers committed more concretely to expanding mental health provision. Deutsch's call for additional funding, then, was not ignored. On the contrary, and as Chapter 4 will illustrate, the US Congress moved to enact the 1963 Community Mental Health Center Act, which provided funds for the construction and expansion of outpatient mental health centers.[5] In contrast to this landmark "bold new approach" heralded by President Kennedy in 1963, the French sectorization policy was born of a mere administrative circular drafted in 1960.[6] In effect, postwar policy-makers in the United States appeared more committed to expanding psychiatric services than their French counterparts, and yet the opposite would eventually occur.

In sum, French and American deinstitutionalization emerged out of broadly similar contexts. In both countries, the end of the Second World

---

there was relatively little effort to support clients who sought to exercise their political voice on their own. The early 20th-century French and American "mental hygiene" movements, for example, aligned themselves with the patient perspective but both were directed by psychiatric professionals (Grob 1983; Henckes 2007).

[4] Moreover, the likelihood of institutionalization in France plummeted from 230.5 in 1935 to 155.3 in 1945 (author's calculations, see Chapter 2). In effect, in 1955 France had only just rebounded from this decline.

[5] Mental Retardation and Community Mental Health Centers Construction Act of 1963, Pub. L. No. 88–164, 77 Stat. 282, codified at 42 U.S.C. ch 33. subch I–V.

[6] John F. Kennedy, "Mental Health Programs: Address to the Congress of the United States," *Journal of the Senate* (February 5, 1963), 108–13.

TABLE 3.2 *Mental health care supply in the United States and France before and after deinstitutionalization*

	1955		1985	
	United States	France	United States	France
Residents per 100,000	338.19	231.72	46.67	145.37
Hospitals per 100,000	0.17	0.22	0.12	0.22

Source: Comparative Deinstitutionalization Data Set (Chapter 2; Appendix)

War was followed by a period of economic growth and welfare state expansion that rendered deinstitutionalization possible. Several factors suggested that the process could have unfolded in a similar way in both countries as well. Fragmented, occupation-based social protection facilitated the transition of elderly residents from mental hospitals and into long-term-care facilities, while care for the poor and destitute mentally ill depended on the generosity of local public authorities. These decentralized government institutions could not count on the powerful medical profession for support, as nonpsychiatric physicians advocated for private sector solutions to health care challenges. Policy elites, however, did have an interest in expanding public services in psychiatry, and even shared a transatlantic vision for reform. A midcentury observer, moreover, might have bet on the Americans' capacity to implement that reform over the French. The United States had developed a firm legislative commitment to expanding community services, while France found itself devastated by the tragic loss of patients during the war. What follows, however, points to one area that would benefit French reform ambitions in ways unavailable to Americans: the possibility for a public labor–management coalition in mental health care.

DIVERGING POSSIBILITIES FOR A PUBLIC LABOR–MANAGEMENT COALITION

Despite these similar initial conditions, public mental health workers in postwar France were much more likely to form a political coalition with their managers than their American counterparts. This difference – the central divergence of the supply-side policy feedback model presented in Chapter 1 (Figure 1.2) – increased the likelihood that France would observe positive supply-side policy feedback in the longer term. Meanwhile, the cards were stacked decidedly against that option in the

United States, where public sector labor unions had not yet gained significant organizational and legal rights to voice their demands. Debilitating workers further, public psychiatric managers organized with private managers, the hypothesized obstruction to this coalition. In France, however, public sector workers gained legal recognition and rights just after the Second World War, and public psychiatric managers organized independently of private managers. The following pages review these chief differences and then addresses potential confounders.

Public Sector Unionization in Postwar America and France

Compared to those of their midcentury French counterparts, the legal and organizational rights of American employees of public mental health services were limited. Although private sector workers had gained collective bargaining rights at the national level in 1935, decisions about those rights for public sector workers were left largely to individual states.[7] As a result, as Alexis Walker (2020, 5) writes, "public sector employees had to fight for legal recognition in every state and locality, which progressed slowly." That the overall trade union movement had suffered under the Taft–Hartley Act in 1947 only weakened the public unionization movement further, even if much of the bill did not directly apply to government workers or their supervisors.[8] Not until the 1960s and 1970s, after deinstitutionalization was well underway, did government employees begin to gain substantial political voice and legislative momentum. Furthermore, as Walker shows, this divided labor law not only repressed the representation of public employees but also weakened the overall trade union movement by fragmenting its membership. American public employees were thus politically weak and therefore absent from discussions about mental health and other social welfare policies in the period immediately following the Second World War.

Although midcentury public sector workers in France faced their own set of complex and varied challenges, many more were able to join unions. As of 1946, these workers could even strike under certain circumstances, a right almost unimaginable to American public employees at the time. As Chapter 5 will explain, mental health workers in France

---

[7] Federal employees, meanwhile, did not gain official recognition until a 1962 Executive Order and, even then, their collective rights would (and still do) vary by agency and work classification. Exec. Order No. 10988, 27 Fed. Reg. 551 (January 19, 1962).

[8] Labor Management Relations Act of 1947 (Taft–Hartley Act), Pub. L. No. 80–101, 61 Stat. 136, codified at 29 U.S.C. ch 7 § § 141–97.

became a more active player in mental health care after 1968, when public employment expanded overall and in outpatient services in particular; however, their access to political voice was far more straightforward than in the United States. In effect, the employees of French public mental health services were better equipped to express their demands to managers throughout the postwar period.

How Public Psychiatric Managers Organized in the United States and France

Meanwhile, if the hypothesis laid out in Chapter 1 is correct, French public psychiatric managers also were better equipped to enter into a coalition with workers than their American counterparts. By the end of the Second World War, French public psychiatric managers had formed a distinctive organization, in fact a trade union itself: the Syndicat des médecins des hôpitaux psychiatriques (i.e., the Syndicat). In contrast, American public psychiatric managers formed just a part of the umbrella American Psychiatric Association (i.e., APA), which included a rapidly growing number of private practitioners. The first organization would help to amplify the political voice of public managers while the second muted it, as subsequent chapters will show (and as I have demonstrated elsewhere, e.g., Perera 2022). This difference would allow the Syndicat to act in accordance with the interests of the public sector more readily than the APA.

The political formation of these two organizations deserves special attention. Unlike the differences in national-level public sector labor rights just outlined, these alternative managerial organizations were particular to mental health care. As such, one might wonder about endogeneity. Did something about the existing mental health system bias American and French managers toward each of these representative institutions? Such concerns are less relevant to differences in public sector labor organization, insofar as the provision of different public services varies within each case (regardless of the overall political strength of their employees). Managerial interests, however, were more explicitly tied to the particularities of mental health care. To that end, scholars have not traditionally interpreted these physician associations as managerial organizations, yet the administration and management of services were (and in many ways still are) a crucial element of psychiatric practice.

Next, I trace the historical development of both the French and American managerial organizations. I draw on both the secondary source histories of the psychiatric profession in each country and primary source statements from the actors themselves. In so doing, several points become clear. First, administration and management have long been a core component of psychiatric practice, especially in the public sector. These economic and political interests, furthermore, shape the politics of the profession in ways underemphasized by the existing historiography. Finally, a series of gradual institutional changes produced the alternative organizational forms. Faced with similar political and economic challenges, actors in each organization adapted differently. Over time, managers in France slowly exerted their independence from private practitioners, even as American managers began to draw closer to private practitioners. This process of "conversion" – wherein new groups are incorporated to an institution and in doing so alter its form, role, and meaning – is especially evident in the American case, in contrast with the evolution of the French case (Mahoney and Thelen 2009; Rocco and Thurston 2014; Thelen 2004).

Both the APA and the Syndicat can trace their roots to the mid 1800s, when the modern psychiatric profession began to emerge. As "alienists" (*aliénistes*), physicians of the mind attended to mental "aliens" (*aliénés*), those patients whose psychological state isolated them from societal functions and norms. Treatment in an "asylum" (*asile*) was thought to ameliorate (or otherwise manage) the condition, so alienists also found themselves directing these proto-hospitals, overseeing their staff, administering their accounts, and, of course, representing their interests to the government authorities who often financed them. The psychiatric profession, in short, was as managerial as it was medical. Over time, alienists would become "psychiatrists," aliens would become "patients," and asylums would become "hospitals," but the link between the profession and public service administration would remain.

That this link emerged during a key moment of modern state formation is no coincidence. Alienists on both sides of the Atlantic were closely aligned with their respective postrevolutionary state-building enterprises. Not only did the new government institution of the asylum provide a secure income for the sons of the emerging *petite bourgeoisie*, the profession itself also offered an identity rooted in science, rationality, and impartiality. Such were the core values of these two newly enlightened republics. Trained in nascent medical schools, alienists soon rejected "spiritualism" (which emphasized the role of spiritual and metaphysical factors on illness) for "science" (which focused primarily on the functions of the body) and instead looked to statistical methods and other emerging technologies to understand both the medical and the managerial aspects of their profession (Dowbiggin 1991; Goldstein 1987; McGovern 1985). In doing so, they also upheld and reinforced state attempts to maintain social order, a central government objective in both the United States and France during the turbulent 19th century.

The organizations representing American and French alienists also identified firmly with the statist side of the major sociopolitical divides of the period. In the United States, an emerging independent bureaucracy sought to counter patterns of heavy-handed patronage (Carpenter 2001; Skowronek 1982). The Association of Medical Superintendents for American Institutions for the Insane (hereafter, the American Superintendents' Association), founded in 1844, defined itself in opposition to these patterns. The appointment of alienists to head insane asylums, they believed, should be based on merit, not partisan connections. The American Superintendents' Association was aware that political skills were crucial to their profession, especially in an environment where bureaucratic imperatives remained subordinate (McGovern 1985, chap. 4). Nonetheless, in 1848 the American Superintendents passed a resolution that "deprecated" attempts to appoint alienists "through political bias," instead backing the "best men irrespective of every other consideration" (quoted in McGovern 1985, 143–44). Aspiring to nonpartisanship and meritocracy, American alienists hence rejected the politics of patronage in lieu of a more Weberian identity.

Meanwhile, in France, a sharp Church/State conflict was seething. Religious authorities oversaw many asylums, which rendered these and many other social services targets for anti-clericalists (see, e.g., Ansell and Lindvall 2020; Morgan 2006). In fact, the 1838 asylum law was a result of this tension. The *Doctrinaires* – a powerful segment of the political elite of the July Monarchy (1830–48) – were critical of the Church's influence on political, social, and economic affairs and sought to establish *département*-level asylums to compete with the religious ones. The move expanded the number of alienists and strengthened their link to the state (Goldstein 1987). For reasons similar to those of their American counterparts, French alienists were beginning to view themselves as rational, scientific, and bureaucratic actors (Dowbiggin 1991). Finding favor among the *Doctrinaires*, the alienists began their first professional association, the Société Médico-Psychologique, in the 1840s. Although both the tumult of the 1848 Revolution and French law restricted their ability to host regular, public meetings, the initial members of the French Société – like their counterparts and frequent interlocuters, the American

Superintendents[9] – also emphasized the profession's managerial, financial, scientific, and public sector orientation (Dowbiggin 1991, chap. 4;
Goldstein 1987, 339–42). Despite their parallel origins, however, the
organizations that represented public sector psychiatric managers in the
United States and France slowly began to evolve in different directions
over the following century.

Between the late 1800s and the Second World War, though, the organizational representation of psychiatric managers evolved differently in
the United States than it did in France. American public managers eventually came to organize together with private practitioners, even though
the original commitment of the American Superintendents' Association
to the public sector was unquestionable. In fact, the group was founded
in part to advocate for state funding of insane asylums, especially those
built according to the therapeutic architecture designed by Dr. Thomas
Kirkbride. The massive "Kirkbride asylums" required a parcel of land
of at least 100 acres and significant government support for their construction.[10] Membership of the Association, furthermore, was restricted
to "medical superintendents," a term that underscored both their clinical and their managerial responsibilities, as well as their predominantly
public employment. Although a few directors of non-state hospitals
requested to join the organization, only one ever served on a committee and only three ever delivered papers at annual meetings in the mid
1800s (McGovern 1985, 136–37). In fact, when Dr. Edward Jarvis delivered a paper in 1860 on "The Proper Functions of Private Institutions or
Homes for the Insane," discussants Dr. D. T. Brown and Dr. MacFarland
observed "very great prejudice" and a "drift of sentiment on the part
of the Association" against "an institution of private character."[11] The
Superintendents' Association, in short, firmly rejected private practice.

Yet, by the late 1800s, as industrialization took hold in the United
States, the Superintendents' Association found itself facing conflict on

[9] A simple review of the cumulative index to SMP's journal, the *Annales Médico-
Psychologiques*, during this period makes the frequency of contact between the two
organizations clear. Leading figures from the American Superintendents (e.g., Dr.
Isaac Ray) and innovative states (e.g., Pennsylvania, Massachusetts) even receive their
own entries. See Baillarger, Cerise, and Lunier, *Annales médico-psychologiques: table
générale et alphabétique 1843–1878* (Paris: Victor Masson et Fils, 1868).

[10] Kirkbride, *On the Construction, Organization, and General Arrangements of Hospitals
for the Insane* (Philadelphia, 1854).

[11] See Jarvis, Brown, and MacFarland in "Proceedings of the Fifteenth Annual Meeting of
the Association of Medical Superintendents of American Institutions for the Insane,"
Journal of Insanity 17–18 (1860), 17–35.

several fronts. Rapid technological development had shifted the structure and orientation of production, reorganizing society with it. The economic crisis of the 1870s had left asylums underfunded as well as overcrowded (Barton 1987). The massive immigration wave of the late 1800s, increasing rates of older patients suffering from senile dementia, and rising numbers of alcoholics and opium addicts expanded the resident population of state hospitals, which lacked the funds to humanely accommodate them (McGovern 1985, 150–51). As the quality of asylum care declined, public criticism increased too. Former asylum patients such as Elizabeth Packard and Clifford Beers became anti-psychiatry and anti-asylum activists, raising the national profile of their abusive experiences and prompting public investigations of asylum conditions (McGovern 1985, 156). These criticisms significantly tarnished the Superintendents' public image, so much so that another organization, the National Association for the Protection of the Insane and Prevention of Insanity, was mounted in direct opposition to them in 1880, though the diversity of opinion among the membership of this rival organization meant it was short-lived (this likely led to its rapid disassociation in 1883).[12]

Neurologists, newly emerged professional and economic competitors, perhaps posed the most important challenge to American alienists. "Your hospitals are not our hospitals; your ways are not our ways," sneered the neurologist S. Weir Mitchell at a turn-of-the-century conference address to the American Superintendents Association. Their specialties, though linked, were in fact different. If the alienists' "real specialty [was] insane-hospital management" for "wretched and neglected" psychotic patients, as one attendee of that conference put it, neurologists specialized in clinical care and research for "nervous diseases" or "neurosis" among the more affluent. The discipline had emerged after the Civil War, when postbellum academic researchers began to investigate the effects of gunshot wounds to the brain and nerve tissues (McGovern 1985, 158; see also Barton 1987, 52–44). By the late 1800s, neurologists had established themselves in urban universities and private offices, catering to a growing patient base from the middle and upper classes (Grob 1994, 50–51; McGovern 1985, 158). Unlike the insanity and psychosis that were prevalent among the poor and destitute living in asylums, nervous diseases

---

[12] *National Association for the Protection of the Insane and the Prevention of Insanity* (Boston: Tolman & White, 1880); *Papers and Proceedings of the National Association for the Protection of the Insane and the Prevention of Insanity, at the Stated Meeting Held in New York City* (New York: G. P. Putnam's Sons, 1882).

were viewed as mild conditions, unthreatening to the social order and more permissible among the upper strata of society. The economic preferences of neurologists therefore were distinct from those of the alienists, a difference underemphasized in the existing historiography, which instead tends to highlight their professional and therapeutic differences. While the alienists required public funds for their profession, neurologists benefited from private affluence.

These interconnected threats of financial strain, public backlash, and the economic competition of neurologists forced the American Superintendents to reconsider their political commitments to public institutions for the poor. How should alienists revamp their image? What alternate sources of funding could support their profession? Should they beat or join their rivals, the neurologists? Responses to these questions emerged slowly, in a series of subtle changes to the organizational rules governing membership of the Superintendents' Association.

Between 1885 and 1921, the Superintendents' Association gradually opened the doors of membership to private practitioners; so much so that, by the middle of the 20th century, private practitioners constituted the overwhelming majority of the Association's members (Grob and Goldman 2006, 17). The first small shift occurred in 1885, when the association changed its membership rules to include assistant physicians, not just the superintendents of public asylums. A younger crop, that had been exposed to neurological training and not yet carrying managerial responsibilities, these new members began to shift discussions at meetings away from administrative concerns and toward more scientific ones (McGovern 1985, 159–61). In 1892, these junior (nonmanagerial and neurologically trained) physicians gained admission, if not the right to vote, in the temporarily renamed "American Medico-Psychological Association" (Grob 1983, 69). Here, too, the composition of attendees and the subjects discussed at annual meetings continued to shift away from the public sector. In time, private practitioners began to attend meetings with the intention of recruiting psychiatrists out of public practice.[13] The organization came to fully embrace this practice, and these new members, by the time it adopted its new name in 1921: the American Psychiatric Association (APA).[14] By 1940, private practitioners composed more than a third of the APA's members. Following an increase

---

[13] Pierce Clark, "Extra Asylum Psychiatry," *American Journal of Insanity* 74 (1918), 425–29.
[14] "Constitution and By-laws," *American Journal of Psychiatry* 78 (1921), 247–52.

in dues, making it difficult for practitioners with lower wages (such as those in the public sector) to join, membership of private practitioners jumped to over 80 percent by the mid 1950s (Grob 1991). As a result, the majority of the mid 20th-century APA was "neither knowledgeable about nor sympathetic toward their institutional brethren" (Grob and Goldman 2006, 17). This stands in sharp contrast to the orientation of its mid 19th-century ancestor, the Superintendents' Association. Now, the interests of the organization's public sector members became secondary, and furthermore these public sector members had no association of their own to join.

In France, meanwhile, alienists faced the same challenges as their American counterparts had in the late 1800s and early 20th century, except their organizational evolution differed. Like the American Superintendents' Association, the Société Médico-Psychologique also initially sought to unite the community of public alienists and represent their economic interests. As the historians Ian Dowbiggin (1991) and Jan Goldstein (1987) have found, publications by key members in the early 1840s made these twin objectives clear (see pages 76–78 and pages 339–41, respectively). The French Société would seek "the improvement of insane asylums," wrote B. A. Morel (1845), and "powerfully promote [these] demands ... to the government in the interest of this unfortunate class of society entrusted to our care," added Honoré Aubanel (1846). Such political-economic ambitions aligned closely with alienists' social-professional identity, for "financial questions ... were the material representation of [alienists'] doctrines," as Émile Renaudin (1846) put it (cited in Dowbiggin 1991, 77 and Goldstein 1987, 340–41, respectively, their translations). Ironically, while the clarity of these commitments among members of the French Société blurred more quickly than they did among members of the American Superintendents, it was French, not American, public psychiatrists who ultimately redefined their independence from private practitioners.

Almost immediately after it was founded, the French Société faced conflicts similar to those of their American counterparts. Following the 1848 Revolution, French alienists lost their liberal, anti-clerical *Doctrinaire* supporters and instead found themselves attempting to appease the more conservative, monarchical Bonapartists. As a result, they faced criticism from both political camps. The political descendants of the *Doctrinaires*, the liberals, launched a massive newspaper campaign that accused alienists of infringing on civil liberties and denounced them as "miserable slaves of power, police assassins" (Regnault cited in Goldstein 1987,

353; translation hers). Meanwhile, the Bonapartists adopted strict surveillance measures to control and repress any suggestion of anti-religious sentiment within the group (Goldstein 1987, 355–56). Such constraints limited the French Société's ability to defend itself and, over the following decades, led to widespread public accusations against the perceived arbitrary incarceration of patients to asylums. Even while this allegation was truer of the profit-seeking private sector than it was of public institutions, it was nevertheless primarily framed as a charge to public sector practitioners (Dowbiggin 1991, 95). That French public asylums, much like American ones, faced financial constraints and overcrowding as industrial production waxed and waned did little to improve their tarnished image (Dowbiggin 1991, 167–68).

In addition, the neurological challenge to public sector alienism was just as forceful in France as it was in the United States. In fact, at the time France was home to the internationally renowned Jean-Martin Charcot, who is still celebrated today as the "founder of modern neurology" (despite his controversial research on hysteria). Charcot (and his circle of fellow students and researchers), much like his American counterparts, tended to practice in urban university centers (especially Paris) and cater to the affluent. The treatment of mild *névroses* (neuroses), furthermore, mainly took place in *maisons de santé* ("health homes"), private clinics where aristocratic families interned their mentally ill relatives (Goldstein 1987, 338).[15] The 1838 law mentioned earlier in this chapter, moreover, had protected these *maisons* precisely to avoid handing "a virtual monopoly over a lucrative market" to the alienists (Goldstein 1987, 400). By the late 1800s, these private sector competitors posed a significant political and economic challenge to the initial public sector identity of the French alienist.

As in the United States, the responses of French public alienists to these challenges involved a series of minor and gradual organizational adjustments. Following the 1848 Revolution, the French Société refounded itself in 1852. This time, its by-laws emphasized scientific purposes over economic ones.[16] To be sure, the Société's membership base remained with the public alienists and generated concern for economic

---

[15] This is not to say that nervous conditions were not diagnosed among the lower class in France. Goldstein (1987, 333–36) cites a study by Briquet, published in 1859, that found that "popular classes were more susceptible to hysteria than their betters." The study helped to supply more clientele to asylums, but after a series of intellectual battles, ultimately failed to associate the study and practice of neurology with the public sector.

[16] *Nouveau règlement de la Société médico-psychologique* (Paris: Martinet, 1852), 3–11.

issues, so much so that it founded an insurance plan for disabled alienists and their widows and orphans (Goldstein 1987, 342). But in principle the Société welcomed the participation of mental scientists from all
disciplines, including neurology. After the Revolution-era legal restrictions on corporatist associations, guilds, and trade unions loosened in
subsequent decades, the Société gained ministerial permission to hold
regular, large public gatherings. According to the available records, the
first "International Conference on Mental Medicine" (Congrès international de médecine mentale) took place in 1878 in Paris.[17] Article 3
of the by-laws of the Congrès notes that its membership was open to
those in the Société but also "all those interested in questions related to
mental alienation," for a reduced fee, no less.[18] After about 1890, the
Société renamed the event the "Conference for French and Francophone
Alienist Physicians and Neurologists" (Congrès des médecins aliénistes et
neurologistes de France et des pays de langue française). By that point,
therefore, public sector alienists and their private sector competitors regularly attended scientific gatherings together, even though their political
organization remained ambiguous.

Over the next two decades, this ambiguity became an increasingly sensitive issue that began to pry open the divide between public and private
practitioners in France. "Dividing the army of workers into two separate
groups, one concerned with nervous conditions and another with mental
illnesses is completely artificial," implored M. Stéhelin, the prefect (head)
of a French *département*, at the 1896 conference. "They should not be
separated," he added.[19] His plea for unity laid bare the tensions between
private physicians of "nervous conditions" and public alienists of "mental illness." In fact, as soon as M. Stéhelin's speech ended, a group of public practitioners left to discuss the subject of creating a Union of French
Alienists.[20] This union did not immediately materialize, for reasons that I

[17] Like the American Superintendents' Association that counted both Americans and
Canadians among their membership, the French Société and its conferences were also
transnational. It often hosted conferences across borders, in cities that included Paris,
Geneva, and Brussels. The fact that the Congrès met in these cities, as well as in France's
smaller capitals such as Bordeaux and Toulouse, is perhaps a sign of both its attempts to
build a cosmopolitan scientific community and its attentiveness to the practical concerns
of provincial alienists.

[18] *Rapports du Congrès internationale de médecine mentale tenu à Paris du 5 au 10 août
1878*, 3.

[19] "Septième session tenue à Nancy du 1er au 5 août 1896," *Comptes rendus du Congrès
des médecins aliénistes et neurologistes de France et des pays de langue française*, 9.

[20] Ibid., 13.

only can speculate. On the one hand, the limited organizational rights of civil servants at the time favored the development of informal *amicales* ("friendly societies") instead of professional associations or trade unions (Siwek-Pouydesseau 1989).[21] On the other hand, the public alienists did not yet face a direct challenge from private practitioners.

By 1907, the situation had changed. Just before that year's conference, the directors of private *maisons de santé* had formed their own group "in defense of their own professional interests."[22] In response, the alienists announced the Association amicale des médecins des établissements publics d'aliénés (Friendly Society of Public Asylum Physicians) with an eight-page spread in the profession's leading journal, the *Annales médico-psychologiques*.[23] Although both groups attended their joint conference, public and private practitioners had now formed separate interest organizations.

While the Société would continue its scientific initiatives and joint conferences of alienists and neurologists, the splintering society of alienists would eventually produce the Syndicat of public psychiatrists over the next half-century. The path was slow and winding. Nicolas Henckes (2007) has documented how the group strengthened and solidified its independent identity in rich detail. For example, he writes about how, during the interwar period, one member, Édouard Toulouse, launched a movement to expand and develop the treatment of milder conditions and neuroses outside of the existing public asylum system, incidentally inspired by the contemporaneous trend in the United States. It took ten years for the friendly society to expel him and clarify its commitments to public practice (Henckes 2007, 148). Toulouse's League for Mental Hygiene, along with an emerging trade union of "nervous system" physicians, would eventually become a chief competitor of the public practitioners (Henckes 2007, 377–80). Later, during the Second

[21] For most of the 19th century, professional associations in France were all but illegal. The 1791 Le Chapelier Law, a product of the first phase of the French Revolution (1789–99), forbade guilds and outlawed the right to strike, in the interest of promoting free enterprise and banishing the *Ancien Régime* practice of corporate favoritism. But even beyond guilds, the Napoleonic Code (effective as of 1804) stipulated government surveillance of any association with more than 20 members. It was not until the latter part of the century that these rules were relaxed, first with the 1884 Loi Waldeck-Rousseau, which authorized working-class unionization. Physician unionization was finally permitted via a more comprehensive law passed in 1892.

[22] "Association amicale des médecins des établissements publics d'aliénés," *Annales Medico-Psychologiques* 5–6 (1907), 221–27.

[23] Ibid.

World War, Nazi occupants forced the friendly society to rename itself the Professional Association of French Psychiatric Hospital Physicians (Association professionnelle des médecins des hôpitaux psychiatriques français). It was not until after the Liberation – and the expansion of public sector organizing rights – that the Syndicat was established in 1947.

Even at this stage, the Syndicat could have reconciled itself to private practitioners and developed an association that resembled the American Psychiatric Association.[24] In fact a leading member of the Syndicat, Georges Daumezon, advocated as much. Between 1945 and 1947, furthermore, the Syndicat contemplated whether it should affiliate with the main medical association, the CSMF. This umbrella organization represented most French physicians, which included many of those in private practice. The French public psychiatrists, however, voted against joining the Confederation. The Syndicat also voted against joining the central, communist-led General Confederation of Labor (Confédération générale du travail, or CGT), as well as the unions and organizations representing civil servants. French public psychiatrists instead sought complete autonomy.[25] Their independent political voice, as Chapter 5 will demonstrate, hence rendered them important partners for public mental health employees in the following decades.

CONFOUNDERS

In sum, by the end of the Second World War, the political economy of mental health in the United States and France shared many similarities, save one key difference. Employees and managers of American public mental health services were far less likely to form a coalition than their French counterparts, who enjoyed both greater legal rights and a unified, independently represented managerial organization. This difference, as shown in subsequent chapters, played a crucial role in the two countries' diverging paths to postwar deinstitutionalization, rendering the United States less likely to expand public mental health services during that period than France. Before moving to that period of diverging paths, however, it is important to consider potential confounders: that is, whether other factors that influenced the likelihood of a coalition could

[24] Georges Daumezon, "L'American Psychiatric Association," *Information psychiatrique* 23:7 (1947), 203.
[25] See the issues of *L'Information psychiatrique* between 1945 and 1947. For a key article on the topic, see P. Sivadon, "Médecins ou fonctionnaires ?," *L'Information psychiatrique* (1946), 7–9.

also have influenced the trajectory of mental health care. Here I consider a few candidates, though none gains enough traction to outweigh the central importance of the public labor–management coalition.

Perhaps France and the United States started off with different rates of public employment and a different propensity toward work in that sector? Did the strong French state simply have more public employees who advocated for unionization earlier there? Not quite. In 1960, total public employment (as a percentage of the working age population) was not significantly higher in France compared to the United States: 11.79 percent and 8.85 percent, respectively (Cusack 2004). It would be difficult to argue that this three-percentage point difference would so radically alter the trajectory of deinstitutionalization in the two countries. Moreover, as Siwek-Pouydesseau (1989, 11) writes, of the one million public employees in postwar France, about a quarter were teachers, not health care workers.

On a related note, it was not necessarily the case that employment in public mental health services was more prestigious in France than it was in the United States. Although it is true that civil service employment in France generally carries great prestige, the employees of public mental health services were not Parisian "fonctionnaires" (bureaucrats). French public psychiatrists in fact complained of the hostility toward their profession.[26] As Henckes (2007) has documented, the social status of those employed in the public mental hospital was far less prestigious than that of the university hospitals or private clinics (331–34). The relative unpopularity of working in French public mental health services, therefore, made it unlikely to drum up the support of its employees for the sake of protecting any perceived prestige.

Turning more specifically to public psychiatric managers, even while the structure of medical interest representation and training may have reinforced the gradual organizational changes made by psychiatrists in the United States and France, it is not clear that it also shaped their mental health policies. Since the 1840s, American medical labor has become more integrated than its fractious French counterpart. In the United States, physicians chose individually whether to affiliate with the primary representative of the medical profession, the American Medical Association (AMA), and/or a specialized representative (in the case of psychiatrists, the APA). This arrangement has not only allowed many

---

[26] G. Daumezon, "Situation actuelle de la psychiatrie, ses perspectives d'avenir," *L'Information psychiatrique* 22:3 (1945), 7–8.

American private sector psychiatrists to elect to join both the APA and the AMA (kindling the political affinity of the two organizations); it has also made it more difficult for American public psychiatrists to establish an independent political voice. But these changes coevolved and in fact cannot be assumed to bias American physicians toward private practice. As Peter Swenson (2021) has shown, the AMA was especially progressive during the early 20th century but later became more conservative. Moreover, the US structure of medical interest representation has not prevented the establishment of some public health services for vulnerable populations, such as Indigenous and veteran Americans.

The development of medical organization and training in France, by contrast, contributed to the isolation of public psychiatrists, if not necessarily the expansion of their services. The confederal structure of French medical labor has resulted in highly factionalized physician interests, often down to very granular levels. A single medical discipline can be broken down into multiple syndicates (representing, for example, academic physicians, subspecialties, salaried physicians, medical students, etc.). Indeed, the French Syndicat is a good example, especially since it was able to exercise its option not to affiliate with the medical confederation. Moreover, French psychiatric education required a period of training at public hospitals. This difference may have contributed to the independent identity of French public psychiatrists; however, and as shown in Chapter 5, they did use the medical training system as a tool to expand public employment – but only after they formed the Syndicat. More importantly, neurologists completed the same training. Unlike many other countries, the disciplines of psychiatry and neurology did not formally split in France until the 1960s, that is, students of each field shared coursework and training. This close association between the two disciplines makes their divided political representation all the more surprising.

Perhaps the most obvious potential confounder is the relative strength of the political Left and labor in general in France compared to the United States. The postwar period hardened this difference. McCarthyism was weakening the American Left precisely as the Liberation sought revenge on Nazi collaborationists on the French Right. But it is not clear how that difference might have shaped public mental health services. As noted in Chapter 1, mental health care does not tend to gain in electoral importance. Political parties and trade unions, therefore, have little reason to advocate for more mental health services (though see Rogers 2022 on how they can shape the philosophy that guides provision). In addition, and as I discussed in the opening of this chapter, the same reformist enthusiasm for more humane treatment existed in both countries.

In Chapters 4 and 5, I turn to this shared blueprint for mental health care reform in both countries. Chapter 4 documents how the absence of a public labor–management coalition in the United States prevented the enactment of mental health care reform and Chapter 5 shows how its presence in France enabled it. Revising standard narratives about the development of psychiatric deinstitutionalization in the United States, I explain why the rise of public employment in America did not manage to maintain its large state mental health infrastructure. On the contrary, the absence of a coalition led to weakening support for these services. Deinstitutionalization proceeded dramatically, with devastating results for people with mental illnesses in that country.

4

Deinstitutionalization in the United States

Why did US policy-makers tear down Allentown State Hospital in 2020? The eventual demolition of that facility, described in Chapter 1, was hardly the intention of their policy-making predecessors in mid 20th-century America. As demonstrated in the preceding chapter, the political and economic conditions of the United States were broadly similar to those of France at the end of the Second World War. As the door to reforming public mental health care opened in earnest, in some ways the United States seemed to have the upper hand. Unlike France, where the war had devastated the supply of mental health services, American mental health care remained in regular use and offered a more robust infrastructure for future expansion, to which US legislators explicitly committed themselves, unlike their counterparts in France. By the early 1960s, Congress had enacted legislation to build a network of 2,000 public outpatient psychiatric clinics. This presented a key first step toward expanding public services for a highly disenfranchised community.

This chapter shows this apparently robust commitment to expanding public mental health care in the United States nonetheless produced the precipitous decline in public mental health service that has since gained notoriety in the international literature on psychiatric deinstitutionalization (e.g., Goodwin 1997; Kritsotaki et al. 2016). Not only did the United States eventually find itself with relatively few public outpatient mental health care services, but the provision of public inpatient care also plummeted. As a result, what was once one of the largest public mental health care systems in the world became one of its smallest (see Figure 1.1). From this influential case, scholars have drawn many conclusions about the process of deinstitutionalization, including its presumed devastating effects on patients. This chapter identifies the political factors that produced such results in the United States, demonstrating how the absence of a public labor–management coalition in mental health produced three negative supply-side policy feedback cycles in the United States. Figures 4.1–4.3 illustrate each cycle in turn, and Table 4.1 at the end of this chapter formalizes how the evidence meets methodological expectations. The repercussions of these cycles have been felt in Allentown and communities like it ever since.

THE FIRST FEEDBACK LOOP: THE STRUGGLES OF PUBLIC COMMUNITY MENTAL HEALTH CENTERS

The end of the Second World War signaled a new era for social reform, including in mental health care. The idea of "community mental health" was among the most popular concepts proposed. This held that a growing number of psychiatric conditions did not require institutional care, and in fact might find better treatment in non-hospital settings, such as outpatient clinics. But who would finance this vision, how, and to what extent? The answers to these questions would shape the viability, size, and patient base of community mental health centers, as well as, crucially, the financial interests of those staffing these centers. The lack of a coalition between public sector managers and workers in postwar America weakened the financial backing of the otherwise "bold new approach" of the 1963 Community Mental Health Center (CMHC) Act. This in turn undermined the ability of the welfare workforce to bolster that backing in the longer term. This first negative supply-side policy feedback loop (Figure 4.1), therefore, placed the outpatient side of psychiatric deinstitutionalization on unstable financial ground.

Public Workers, Managers, and Community Mental Health

In the 1950s and early 1960s, neither public sector workers nor managers were well-positioned to form an alliance on public mental health care in the United States. Public sector trade unions, as noted in Chapter 3, faced numerous organizational and legal challenges in the American states and hence lacked sufficient political power at either the local or federal levels to advocate for the expansion of public employment in mental health. The superintendents of public mental hospitals, meanwhile, lacked an independent political organization. Rather, the American Psychiatric Association (APA) to which they belonged had all but removed public mental hospitals from its political agenda. By the 1950s, more than 80 percent of the

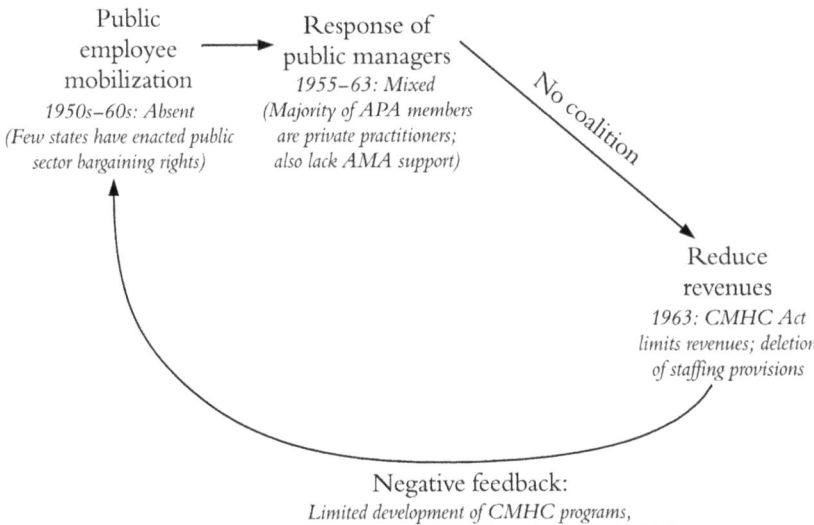

Public
employee
mobilization
1950s–60s: Absent
(Few states have enacted public
sector bargaining rights)

Response of
public managers
1955–63: Mixed
(Majority of APA members
are private practitioners;
also lack AMA support)

No coalition

Reduce
revenues
1963: CMHC Act
limits revenues; deletion
of staffing provisions

Negative feedback:
Limited development of CMHC programs,
whose employees turn to more affluent clients (not public funds) for revenues

FIGURE 4.1 First supply-side policy feedback loop, postwar US mental health care

APA's membership was employed outside of mental institutions (Grob and Goldman 2006, 17). It is no surprise, then, that the voices that most influenced policy discussions about community mental health preferred private sector approaches to implementing the CMHC's "bold new approach."

The political development of the 1955 Joint Commission of Mental Illness and Health is a case in point. The commission resulted from more than a decade of growing federal investment in psychiatric medical and services research (itself in part a product of lobbying from elite researchers in private practice and universities) (Grob 1994). Emboldened by these investments, the APA proposed a new research study: an examination of the "breakdown crisis" of overcrowded, ineffective, and under-resourced postwar state mental hospitals. Supported by its sister organization of private practitioners (the American Medical Association), the APA gained congressional authorization to establish the Joint Commission to both diagnose the problems of the mental health system and develop a program of improvement. Although the commission would include representatives from the APA and the American Medical Association, no public sector trade union participated.[1]

The orientation of the Joint Commission of Mental Illness and Health toward private sector interests did not insulate it from conflict. From its

---

[1] Nor, for that matter, did any organization devoted exclusively to representing clients of mental health services.

small and struggling headquarters in Wisconsin, the American Federation of State, County, and Municipal Employees (AFSCME) had expressed reservations about the influence of the private "medical lobby" on public health provision, though it did applaud the appointment of a former Massachusetts administrator, Dr. Jack R. Ewalt, to head the commission. This support was motivated by the hope that he might sympathize with the public sector cause (RL Publications 26/5; RL Zander Records 8/5). Ultimately, the recommendations proposed by Dr. Ewalt and the commission roiled government employees. The Joint Commission's 1961 report *Action for Mental Health* proposed to ban the construction of state mental hospitals with more than 1,000 beds and to build a network of community clinics to reduce the need for lengthy and recurrent hospitalization. Although the report did call for more federal involvement in financing mental health care, it did not specify whether the community clinics should be private or public, leaving the answer to that important question up for grabs.

"Vociferous criticism" from state mental hospital employees followed (Grob 1991, 212). At a 1961 meeting, government-employed psychiatrists denounced the report's "opinions and biases" in favor of private practice (Grob 1991, 212). Newton Bigelow, a leading New York state hospital official, wrote a series of editorials in *Psychiatric Quarterly* enumerating these complaints. He highlighted both the role that mental hospitals played in caring for the chronically ill and the "real problem" of staff–patient ratios as the cause of ill-treatment in those hospitals. Expanding support for public sector staff, he argued, was the better way to improve mental health care. Nonetheless, the commission's recommendations received a formal stamp of approval from the American Psychiatric Association, as well as the American Medical Association. Indeed their members were the report's primary authors, and they had been especially responsive to private practitioners in their recommendations (Grob 1994, 214).

The 1963 Act Limits Public Revenues for Community Mental Health Centers

Drawing on the formalized (if contentious) recommendations of the Joint Commission, Congress enacted the Mental Retardation and Community Mental Health Centers Construction Act in 1963.[2] John F. Kennedy, then

---

[2] Mental Retardation and Community Mental Health Centers Construction Act of 1963 (Community Mental Health Act), Pub. L. No. 88–164, 77 Stat. 282, codified at 42 U.S.C. ch 33. subch I–V.

president, hailed it as a "bold new approach" to American mental health policy.[3] In reality, its symbolic value may have been more significant than its practical effect. First, its content was vague, as "state, local, and private action" was identified to stimulate the vast array of recommendations. Second, its financial support for public mental health care was weak. Title II of the Act supported, but did not mandate, the construction of the Joint Commission's proposed "public and other nonprofit community mental health centers." No provisions were made to identify the concrete responsibilities of the "CMHCs," nor were the funds allocated to them very large. The federal government expected states to cover a significant portion (one-third to two-thirds) of CMHC construction costs and capped the available national funds at $150 million (about $1.5 million contemporary USD; per BLS 2023) over a restricted three-year period (fiscal years 1965–67). Moreover, the appropriations that would go to academic research – not the delivery of care – took priority. Third, for strategic political reasons, the Act's primary focus was on childhood developmental disabilities, not adult chronic and severe mental illness. Action on the former tended to yield more political support than the latter, which did not benefit from the advocacy of concerned middle- and upper-class parents. In fact, President Kennedy's own family, which sought to redress the challenges faced by his disabled younger sister, Rosemary, helped to promote the Act.

Perhaps the most glaring omission in the 1963 Act was the absence of support for CMHC staff. The private practitioners of the American Medical Association had campaigned intensely to prevent the allocation of federal funds to items beyond construction, especially to personnel costs. Funding staff, the private practitioners expected, would promote the development of a public mental health workforce.[4] Not all of the American Medical Association members opposed the staffing provisions. Initially, it was only its Council on Legislative Activities that strongly criticized the allocation of public funds for CMHC personnel. Its Council on Mental Health, meanwhile, was somewhat more supportive of funding personnel. But in June 1963, its House of Delegates – an elected general assembly that reflected the American Medical Association's private sector majority – voted to disapprove

---

[3] John F. Kennedy, "Mental Health Programs: Address to the Congress of the United States," *Journal of the Senate* (February 5, 1963), 108–13.

[4] In this way, the private practitioners of the American Medical Association adopted the reverse strategy of the public practitioners in the Syndicat in 1968, as shown in the next chapter. Both groups knew that public workers depended on public funds, whose expansion would therefore challenge the American Medical Association and benefit the Syndicat. The two different organizations acted accordingly.

the Act. Conservatives in the congressional House of Representatives seized the opportunity to delete the staffing provisions (Foley 1975, 67–69; Gillon 2000, 95; Grob 1991, 231).

Caught between their public sector minority and private sector majority, as well as their close affiliation with the American Medical Association, the APA did little to protest the deletion of the staffing provisions from the Act. The APA's threadbare presence at the July hearing of the bill, just one month after the American Medical Association's House of Delegates overturned a key provision, indicates just how unimportant the issue was to this organization that served as the primary representative of psychiatric managers. Dr. Ewalt did testify at the hearing, first and foremost in his capacity as a community mental health expert (and not in his capacity as a representative of the APA). When asked about the APA's formal position on the bill, Ewalt noted that it did support the bill and reminded the subcommittee that the American Medical Association had also cosponsored one of the studies that had inspired it.[5] But there was no attempt to underscore the importance of the staffing provisions, by Ewalt or any other APA members at the hearings.

The APA's attitude toward the deletion of the staffing provisions was one of tacit permission. Had public managers in the organization formed a coalition with their employees, perhaps they would have supported these staffing provisions more forcefully, for this was precisely the kind of policy that would have bolstered public employment. But the mixed representation of the APA led the organization to develop a closer relationship with private practitioners in the AMA than with public employees. The APA appears to have traded its silence on public policies that benefit public employees for the AMA's support for public policies that benefit private practitioners. Although in theory the APA could have supported both sets of policies, in practice the cross-pressures led the organization to make strategic choices. Strengthening its support for private practice (over public practice) maximized its chances of policy success on the dimensions most relevant to its membership and primary coalition partner. As a result, the 1963 Act offered a vague blueprint for the expansion of community mental health services, but it was tilted against a lack of stable public financing and, by extension, lack of support for public mental health workers.

---

[5] *Mental Health (Supplemental): Hearings on S.1576, Day 1, Before the Subcommittee of the Committee on Interstate and Foreign Commerce House of Representative.* 88th Cong. 78–79 (1963) (statement of Dr. Jack Ewalt, Former Commissioner, Department of Mental Hygiene, State of Massachusetts, and presently President of the American Psychiatric Association and Superintendent of Massachusetts Mental Health Center).

Negative Feedback in Staffing Provisions

"The real question," an internal memorandum of the Bureau of the Budget observed, "is who is going to finance operating costs [of the CMHCs] once the federal subsidies are ended" (Grob 1991, 230). Although enactment of the 1963 Act did help to construct about 200 community mental health centers, federal administrators became aware that the program could not remain afloat (let alone reach the target of 2,000 centers) without significant, and stable, public financing (Foley 1975, chap. 5; Grob 1991, chap. 10). At first, legislators threw these centers a lifeline: Over the next three years, the Democratic Congress authorized about $700 million for the centers' operational expenses.[6] But this support was short-lived. Moreover, the centers that received support in the first year would receive substantially less in the second and third years (75 percent and 30 percent of the initial amount, respectively) (Grob 1991, 249).

Employees of the CMHCs nonetheless began to advocate for the bill's reauthorization in subsequent years. Although the primary trade union representing public employees (AFSCME) did not formally participate, labor's umbrella organization (the American Federation of Labor and Congress of Industrial Organizations, or AFL-CIO) agreed to coordinate lobbying activities for the bill's reauthorization (Foley 1975, 106). The AFL-CIO viewed the community mental health centers not only as opportunities for employment but also as a social program that might benefit their members.[7] Involved in these lobbying activities, moreover, was the APA, whose recent leadership changes had revived some attention to public practice. Moreover, the American Medical Association had agreed to temper its opposition to the CMHC staffing grants in exchange for the APA's support on other issues of interest to private sector specialists.[8]

---

[6] In contemporary USD (per BLS 2023).

[7] *Research Facilities, Mental Health Staffing, Continuation of Health Programs, and Group Practice: Hearings on HR 2084, HR 2085, HR 2988, HR 2987, Day 4, Before the Committee on Interstate and Foreign Commerce.* 89th Cong. 284–99 (1965) (statement of Lisbeth Bamberger, Assistant Director, Social Security Department, AFL-CIO).

[8] The American Medical Association still voiced their opposition at the bill's hearing, but only briefly, before returning their attention to other bills (on financing the construction of medical and dental group practices). *Research Facilities, Mental Health Staffing, Continuation of Health Programs, and Group Practice: Hearings on HR 2084, HR 2085, HR 2988, HR 2987, Day 4, Before the Committee on Interstate and Foreign Commerce.* 89th Cong. 284–99 (1965) (statement of Lisbeth Bamberger, Assistant Director, Social Security Department, AFL-CIO); also Foley (1975, 108).

Nevertheless, the APA still did not explicitly back public community mental health care during the reauthorization hearings. Speaking on behalf of the Association, Vice President Dr. Addison M. Duval allowed for some conflation of community care and private outpatient practice. Insisting that his colleagues had not been "sitting on [their] hands waiting for a handout from Congress," he instead hailed how "two out of every three mental patients are being treated on an outpatient basis and the majority of them in the private sector of medicine."[9] What he was suggesting, of course, was that Congress should do more to support community care by devoting public funds to it. After all, Dr. Duval was Georgia's Director of the Division of Mental Health and a former employee of the federally funded St. Elizabeth's Hospital in Washington, DC. But he was equally aware that most of his colleagues were uninterested in public practice. "Our task," he offered, "is to help ensure that an ever-greater percentage of [young psychiatrists] will turn from interest in private practice to a broader application of their clinical skills in comprehensive community services."[10] The language of "community," "broad application," and "outpatient basis" carefully avoided any explicit advocacy by the APA on behalf of public service workers. In fact, by distancing CMHCs from state hospitals, the APA loosened the association of mental health care with public sector provision. What is more, eventually the APA "recommended that the [CMHC] staffing grant program be changed to an operational grant program."[11] This more muted language would allow for greater program "flexibility" and kept the concerns of private practitioners at bay by couching any support for public workers in more general language.

Absent a robust coalition between public mental health workers and managers, the staffing grants thus depended on congressional approval.

[9] *Research Facilities, Mental Health Staffing, Continuation of Health Programs, and Group Practice: Hearings on HR 2084, HR 2085, HR 2988, HR 2987, Day 4, Before the Committee on Interstate and Foreign Commerce.* 89th Cong. 204–5 (1965) (statement of Dr. Addison M. Duval, Vice President and Councilor, American Psychiatric Association).

[10] *Research Facilities, Mental Health Staffing, Continuation of Health Programs, and Group Practice: Hearings on HR 2084, HR 2085, HR 2988, HR 2987, Day 4, Before the Committee on Interstate and Foreign Commerce.* 89th Cong. 205 (1965) (statement of Dr. Addison M. Duval, Vice President and Councilor, American Psychiatric Association).

[11] *Physician Training Facilities and Health Maintenance Organizations: Hearings on S. 935, S. 703, S. 837, S. 1182, S. 1301, S. 2827, S. 3327 (Part 6), Day 1, Before the Subcommittee on Health of the Committee on Labor and Public Welfare.* 92nd Cong. 2208 (1972) (statement of Dr. Alfred Freedman, President-Elect, American Psychiatric Association).

Although CMHC employees could expect a Democratic Congress and president to reauthorize the funds for most of the 1960s, the Republican administrations that followed made that possibility less likely. A pattern emerged under America's divided government of the 1970s. A Democratic Congress would renew the CMHC staffing provisions for another three-year term, the Republican president (Nixon, then Ford) would veto the bill, and Congress would override it. But the situation remained tenuous, so much so that it once required legal action. Claiming that the program was never intended as more than a demonstration grant, President Nixon's health secretary, Casper Weinberger, impounded the CMHC funds. But the Democratic Congress protested the move, prompting D.C. District Court judge Gerhard Gesell to overturn the decision and order the funds released (Foley 1975, 130; Grob and Goldman 2006, 62–63).

As the negative feedback continued, CMHC employees began to look elsewhere for funding. Without the regular, sustained, and widespread support of managers, they rarely garnered sufficient state and local funds to make up the difference from insufficient congressional grants. As a result, CMHCs found themselves depending on privately paying patients, for only they could afford the regular, lengthy therapy sessions offered by the centers. As one therapist remarked, CMHCs "began to focus on reaching more clients who could verbalize their problems – and who could pay" (cited in Gillon 2000, 101). Moreover, Congress eventually expanded the community mental health mandate to include services for people experiencing substance abuse and addiction, and for children. In effect, Congress shifted emphasis on serving groups with less intensive, and therefore less costly, needs than those of people with chronic and severe mental illness (Foley 1975, 126; Gillon 2000, 101). This shift meant replacing services intended for the seriously mentally ill (access to medical care, housing, employment) with services for those with milder conditions (marriage counseling, family therapy).

In fact, the demographic shift in the CMHC population was so pronounced that analysts coined an acronym for its new clientele, YAVIS: young, attractive, verbal, intelligent, and successful (Schofield 1964, 133).[12] Very few CMHC patients had severe needs, let alone needs that

---

[12] This acronym, first developed by Schofield, soon became a political weapon for public employees advocating against the privatization of mental health care; see, for example, Jerry Wurf's September 1975 speech to the American Psychiatric Association's Institute on Hospital and Community Psychiatry, "A Worker's View of Mental Health Care" (WF CWS, 1/113, 9).

had required hospitalization.[13] At first, CMHC patients tended to be from poorer and non-white backgrounds, at least in urban areas. But as the first negative feedback loop played out over the next few years, only 15 percent of the total CMHC patient population would fall under the schizophrenic category, the condition that most strained public budgets (Grob 1991, 261; Grob and Goldman 2006, 47). As CMHC employees turned to private revenue sources to preserve their employment, poor patients with severe mental illness were beginning to fall through the cracks.[14]

THE SECOND FEEDBACK LOOP: THE EXCLUSION OF PUBLIC MENTAL HOSPITALS FROM THE SOCIAL SECURITY AMENDMENTS

While negative supply-side policy feedbacks constrained the supply of public community mental health centers, another set of negative feedbacks reduced the supply of state and county mental hospitals (Figure 4.2), the main public providers of inpatient psychiatric care. On average, states allocated nearly a tenth of their overall annual budgets to paying for these facilities.[15] The situation changed in 1965 with the landmark enactment of the Social Security Amendments. This major federal intervention in health and social welfare policy nonetheless excluded state and county mental hospitals. In doing so, it shifted the financial incentives of states by facilitating the transfer of patients out of the hospital setting. In some cases, former psychiatric patients entered private elderly care homes; younger patients did not have that option. The result was a gradual decline in both patient numbers and, by extension, revenues

---

[13] The APA itself acknowledged this. A Joint Information Service study published in 1969 found that five out of eight centers evaluated did little to reduce hospital admissions in their catchment areas (Grob 1991, 255).

[14] The emergence of YAVIS clients also illustrates how the expanding definition of mental health shaped service distribution over time. This new group was politically different from those with severe and chronic needs: YAVIS clients required different services (e.g., more talk therapy but less housing support), were more willing and able to pay for these services out-of-pocket, and relatedly, tended to be more active voters. In other words, the YAVIS political constituency became distinct from those with chronic conditions, competing for policy attention and enabling the development of private (not public) services.

[15] About 8 percent in 1951, though it was less in some states (as little as 2 percent) and much higher in others. In New York, a third of state spending went to mental hospitals (Grob 1991, 161).

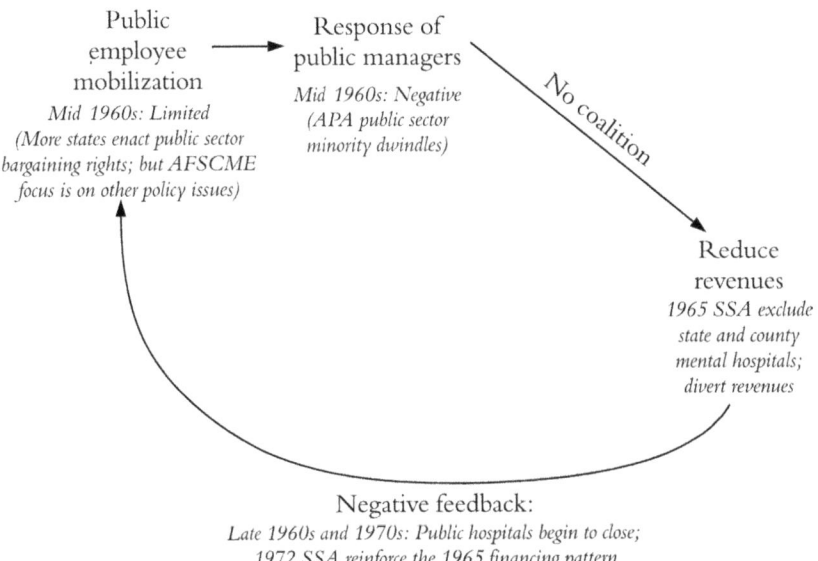

FIGURE 4.2 Second supply-side policy feedback loop, postwar US mental health care

of state and county mental hospitals through the late 1960s and 1970s. Although state public employees had begun to pick up political and legal momentum at this time, they lacked the necessary support of their managers to demand that the Social Security programs expand coverage to mental hospitals.

Moreover, the negative feedback loop rendered them unable to prevent the 1972 enactment of disability insurance from further exacerbating this problem. Long-term public hospital patients, already excluded from the 1965 Medicare and Medicaid programs, then became unable to access disability benefits. Thus, the absence of a coalition between public mental health care workers and managers reduced the availability of federal funds for their patients and, accordingly, their services.

Public Workers, Managers, and Hospitals

Although a select number of states had begun to grant legal rights to organize to their employees by the mid 1960s, the vast majority of employees in state and county mental hospitals remained unorganized at this time. In general, their perspective was absent from the debates on the Social Security Amendments. The American Federation of State, County, and

Municipal Employees did signal an interest in the bill in a letter to the congressional Committee on Ways and Means, but it did not explore – or perhaps was even unaware of – its implications for current state hospital employees.[16] Following the general lead of the AFL-CIO, the small and locally fragmented AFSCME instead focused its attention on the bill's implications for aging workers. The adoption of federal pension and health insurance programs would reduce the union's own obligations to provide these benefits to their members.

While state employees were too unorganized to advocate for public mental hospitals in the bill, the APA focused its efforts on using the bill to support private psychiatric practice. By then, one of the APA's presidents had publicly stated that the state mental hospital was "antiquated, outmoded, and rapidly becoming obsolete" (Grob 1994, 223). Although a small minority of public psychiatrists in the organization protested this image, the APA did little to redress it. Instead, the organization sought to include private psychiatric services in the basket of elderly care benefits provided by the generous new Medicare program. Moreover, the APA's focus was on private outpatient services. It did little to prevent legislators from curtailing Medicare coverage of public inpatient psychiatry, which may have benefited the state and county mental hospitals. In fact, as one APA representative testified, "other types of facilities [than state hospitals] can often render more appropriate treatment at far lower cost – private psychiatric hospitals, day hospitals, outpatient departments, community mental health centers, and so on." The APA unofficially but effectively estranged private practice from public psychiatry to draw greater resources to the private sector at the expense of the public sector.

The 1965 Social Security Amendments Exclude State and County Mental Hospitals

The absence of a coalition between the workers and managers of state and county mental hospitals facilitated the exclusion of these services from the 1965 Social Security Amendments and subsequent legislation. First, the headline Medicare health insurance program and expanded Social Security pension program dramatically reduced the population of elderly

---

[16] *Health Services for the Aged under the Social Security Insurance System: Hearings on H.R. 4222.* 87th Cong. 1979–80 (1961) (Letter from Arnold S. Zander, International President of the American Federation of State, County, and Municipal Employees, AFL-CIO).

patients living in state and county hospitals. Prior to the Amendments' enactment, about one out of every three persons admitted to a mental hospital was over 60 years old, a proportion that had increased by 40 percent in the preceding two decades, as rising female labor force participation and the baby boom challenged the possibility of domestic elderly caregiving.[17] The Medicare program offered elderly Americans health coverage, including in the area of private outpatient psychiatry (due in part to the advocacy of the APA), though it limited the total number of days they could spend as hospital inpatients to 190 days (in their lifetime). Moreover, elderly residents could use the resources offered by the expanded pension, Social Security, to obtain other services. Consequently, Medicare incentivized elderly patients to seek medical coverage outside of the state and county hospital, while Social Security supported their access to alternative custodial care.

Second, Medicaid precluded covering services provided in "institutions for mental disease" (IMDs), which further motivated states to transfer their indigent patients out of state and county mental hospitals. As Laura Katz Olson has detailed, the Medicaid program was an "afterthought" to the 1965 Social Security Amendments, "slipped in" by Wilbur Mills (D-AR) to provide health insurance for the blind, the disabled, and families participating in the Aid to Families with Dependent Children program (Katz Olson 2010, 22–27).[18] Needy patients in mental hospitals were likely to qualify for the new Medicaid program. At the state level, governors and administrators welcomed the opportunity to share the costs of those patients with the federal government, but at the federal level, few in Congress were willing to take on these costs. "When we get into this field [of mental health care] it is going to cost a lot of money," said Senator Russell Long (D-LA).[19] Facing no resistance from the welfare workforce, Congress thus easily excluded IMD payments from the basket of Medicaid benefits (hereafter, the IMD Exclusion). Senator Long's reasoning, moreover, made it difficult for federal policy-makers to include extensive noninstitutional care

---

[17] Action for the Aged and Aging, S. Rep. 128, at 4 (1961).

[18] Over time, Medicaid would become the primary source of health coverage for the poor, but this was not the intention in 1965. In fact, the Amendments restricted coverage by requiring states to share some of the costs of the program (a financial disincentive, especially to the neediest states) and by giving them significant leeway over the scope of coverage (Katz Olson 2010).

[19] *Social Security: Hearings on H.R. 6675, Day 7, Before the Committee on Finance.* 89th Cong. 725 (1965) (statement of Sen. Long).

in the benefit structure of either Medicaid or Medicare. Again facing no resistance from the welfare workforce, Congress presumed that states would continue to provide mental health care services, inpatient and outpatient, on their own dime for the foreseeable future.

Third, Congress enacted a small piece of pork barrel legislation on the heels of the 1965 Amendments that effectively subsidized state mental hospitals' competitors: private elderly care homes by tweaking the federal tax code. The technical and complex bill went through numerous twists and turns, seemingly unnoticed by those in the mental health field (let alone the general public, for that matter). The bill first emerged in the House in March 1965, sponsored by Representative John Byrnes, a Republican from Wisconsin, where a recent survey had found a "serious shortage" of facilities.[20] Although temporarily overshadowed by the Social Security Amendments, the proposal then reappeared in the Senate in September 1966 when Senator Jack Miller (R-IA), of the Committee on Aging, tacked it onto a bill intended to control the costs of tax collection (the IRS had recently implemented a new automatic data processing system). The addition of Section 7, on nursing homes, to the bill would "save the taxpayers several million dollars," his colleague Senator Long assured.[21] At that point, there was enough general agreement among the senators to pass the bill and send it to the House. A joint committee then developed more specific conditions about the "modest profit" available to nursing homes.[22] It stipulated that profits would depend not only on services delivered but also on the costs spent on buildings and construction. Reimbursing based on a reasonable charge instead of a reasonable cost, furthermore, would incentivize both private for-profit and private not-for-profit services to build new nursing homes. Public nursing homes were excluded since they were not driven by the profit motive. On November 2, 1966, President Johnson assented, signing legislation "requiring the Department of Health, Education, and Welfare to permit the nursing homes a modest profit when reimbursing them for their services to Medicare patients."[23] This seemingly small policy

---

[20] Cong. Rec. H28220 (daily ed. October 20, 1966) (statement of Rep. Byrnes).

[21] Cong. Rec. S23644 (daily ed. September 22, 1966) (statement of Sen. Long).

[22] Reimbursement for Proprietary Extended Care Facilities under Medicare, H.R. Rep. 2317 (1966) (Conf. Rep.).

[23] An Act to Amend the Internal Revenue Code of 1954 to Promote Savings under the Internal Revenue Service's Automatic Data Processing System (part of the Older Americans Act of 1965), Pub. L. No. 89–713, 79 Stat. 218 § (1966). codified at 42 U.S.C. ch 35 § § 3001 et seq.

change delivered significant rewards to private elderly care homes, but not state and county mental hospitals.

Negative Feedback in the 1972 Social Security Amendments

The American states henceforth took advantage of these policy changes to reduce their hefty budget lines for public mental hospitals. The federal government's affirmative support for private nursing home care and private psychiatric benefits, combined with its refusal to cover care provided in public institutions, deinstitutionalized the elderly out of mental hospitals and into care homes. Between 1965 and 1972, the rate of admission of individuals over 65 to state and county mental hospitals fell by half, from 146 per 100,000 to 69 per 100,000. The locus of care for these individuals thus shifted from asylums to nursing homes: Between 1960 and 1970, the number of nursing home facilities increased by 140 percent, of nursing home beds by 232 percent, and of nursing home patients by 210 percent (Gillon 2000, 103). Although this shift away from state and county mental hospitals was especially pronounced among the elderly population, Medicaid's IMD Exclusion had also begun to incentivize the deinstitutionalization of younger indigent patients.

As a result of this evolution, the revenues of state and county mental hospitals declined sharply, weakening their workforce further. Moreover, managerial representatives continued their estrangement from the public sector. The APA's positions had evolved: It began taking a stronger stance against Medicare's 190-day limit on inpatient treatment, as well as in favor of lowering coinsurance costs for Medicare outpatients and expanding Medicaid coverage of mental health services in private general hospitals.[24] Lengthening the duration of Medicare coverage for inpatient treatment would benefit private psychiatric and general hospitals; lowering coinsurance costs for outpatient care would benefit clinicians in private offices; and the removal of Medicaid restrictions for poor patients in general hospitals would reduce the volume of care in state and county mental hospitals. Although it had somewhat adjusted its policy positions, the APA supported policies that benefited the majority of its members, those in private practice, and did little to support the minority of its public practitioner members.

---

[24] *Social Security Amendments of 1971: Hearings on H.R. 1, Volume 5, Before the Committee on Finance.* 92nd Cong. 2409 (1972) (statement of Dr. Robert W. Gibson, Medical Director, The Sheppard and Enoch Pratt Hospital, Townson, MD, on behalf of the American Psychiatric Association).

By the early 1970s, there was little the welfare workforce was able to do to prevent federal legislation from repeating the pattern it set forth in the 1965 Social Security Amendments. The 1972 Social Security Amendments – which replaced state welfare programs for the aged, the poor, the blind, and crucially, the disabled with the federally administered Supplemental Security Income program – also excluded payments to people residing in state and county mental hospitals (and indeed, in public institutions more generally, for similar cost-control reasons).[25] Records show no indication that either AFSCME or the APA expected the eligibility exclusion, in part because both groups were more concerned with the bill's immediate implications for their members. The union's narrow focus was on how the possible "federalization" of welfare might displace local social service employees, not on the effects of the bill for psychiatric patients served by state and county hospital employees.[26] Expanding Social Security Disability Insurance (SSDI) benefits to include those in public institutions, in its view, would have little immediate effect on the livelihood of its members. This 1972 policy thus encouraged states to also transfer disabled patients out of state and county mental hospitals. The year following the program's enactment saw a record reduction in the institutionalized population: 13.3 percent (Gillon 2000, 103).

The negative policy feedback that resulted impacted not only the employees of state hospitals but also their patients. Although the relocation of deinstitutionalized patients was a shrewd financial move for the states, it was far from benevolent. A few "psychiatric ghettos" arose in urban centers near deinstitutionalizing hospitals, primarily for the indigent Medicaid patients who lacked a custodial alternative.[27] That many

---

[25] As Erkulwater (2006, 66) has shown, "the passage of SSI had almost nothing to do with the disabled." Instead, it was a political compromise between congressional Democrats and Republicans. While Democrats sought to relieve old-age poverty, Republicans refused to do so through the standard Social Security program (as this would increase spending on all retirees, not just the elderly poor). Client advocates did not play a major role in the program's enactment. Once enacted, however, the program did benefit a section of the disability rights movement, if not as much the mentally ill. Disability advocacy is no stranger to intersectionality. Clients with somatic conditions tend to have better means of expressing their demands to the government than low-income people with long-term and severe mental illness. Moreover, they tend to be most successful at gaining legal rights, rather than securing long-term and generous financing for services.

[26] *Social Security Amendments of 1971: Hearings on H.R. 1, Volume 4, Before the Committee on Finance.* 92nd Cong. 1767 (1972) (statement of Paul J. Minarchenko, Director of Legislation, American Federation of State, County, and Municipal Employees, AFL-CIO).

[27] In 1970, there were approximately 170 halfway houses serving about 3,000 individuals (Grob 1991, 251).

of these patients were eligible now for disability benefits (as long as they did not reenter the institution) reinforced these trends. As private entrepreneurs converted run-down hotels and houses into boarding homes and halfway houses, former mental patients often found themselves living together once again, but this time without professional medical attention. A study in New York City shortly after the passage of the 1972 Amendments found that one in four residents of the city's "welfare hotels" once resided in a public mental hospital.[28]

The elderly patients who now lived in nursing homes, moreover, were not much better off either. Soon enough, about half of nursing home residents were living in cramped facilities with more than 100 beds, and about a third of those patients in facilities with more than 200 beds. The majority of these facilities lacked trained medical staff and few offered the psychiatric care necessary for those with serious conditions (Gillon 2000, 102–3). What had occurred was not the deinstitutionalization of patients from the hospital into the community but rather the transinstitutionalization of patients from a medical institution to a merely custodial one, if they could find one.

THE THIRD FEEDBACK LOOP: THE FORMAL RETRENCHMENT OF PUBLIC MENTAL HEALTH SERVICES

By the early 1970s, the first and second feedback loops had placed severe financial strain on public mental health services. First, only about 400 (out of the projected 2,000) CMHCs had received federal funding.[29] Not only was there dwindling political support for the reauthorization grants but neither had the enactment of Medicare and Medicaid offered much additional support. States were responsible for determining Medicaid reimbursement rates for CMHCs, and Medicare had not given the

---

[28] Some halfway houses received funding from State Divisions of Vocational Rehabilitation (and, by extension, the federal government, which reimbursed up to 80 percent of costs), and rents and fees often depended on patient's disability payments. As a result, most houses relied on private sources of support (from nonprofit and grant-making organizations). This of course garnered little political attention from the for-profit psychiatric workforce. As Raymond Glasscote noted in his study of rehabilitation for the APA at that time, "Many mental health professionals do not have much knowledge of, interest in, or commitment to the importance of rehabilitative and supporting resources that must be available on an intermediate or long-term basis to the seriously ill people that they seek to retain in the community" (ibid.; for the study, see Gillon 2000, 103).

[29] *Extend Community Mental Health Centers Act: Hearing on H.R. 16676, Before the Subcommittee on Public Health and Environment of the Committee on Interstate and Foreign Commerce.* 92nd Cong. 1 (1972).

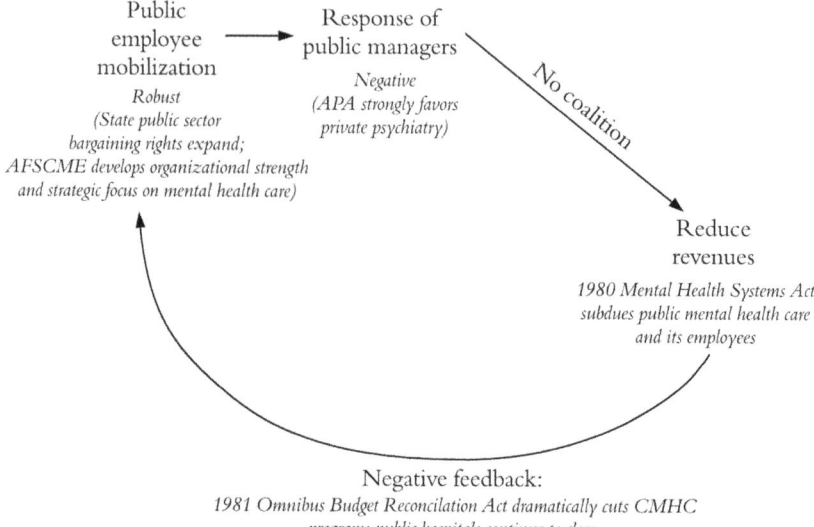

FIGURE 4.3 Third supply-side policy feedback loop, postwar US mental health care

centers the status of designated (covered) provider (PCMH 1978, 31). Second, the deinstitutionalization of state and county mental hospitals had reduced revenues to the point that many states now considered closing their hospitals wholesale. That the scandalous conditions in these underfunded institutions had reached the public's ears only exacerbated the pressure to close hospitals.

In addition to these domestic policy pressures, public mental health services also faced financial strain from international factors. The economic shocks of the early 1970s had prompted governments to scale back their public budgets. The ongoing war in Vietnam, moreover, motivated American officials to withdraw funding from mental health and other social welfare initiatives and instead devote it to defense and military operations (Gillon 2000, 98). In short, public mental health services – and their employees – were facing financial pressures on multiple fronts.

The third negative feedback cycle (Figure 4.3) resulted in the formal retrenchment of public mental health services, both inpatient and outpatient. What is different about this third feedback loop is that public sector workers, now more robustly unionized at the state level, took on a much more active role in resisting these pressures than they had when contending with the first two feedback loops. Nonetheless, workers were unable to form an alliance with their managers, who remained beholden to the representation of the private-oriented American Psychiatric Association. The absence of such a coalition rendered the welfare workforce much less capable of renewing and expanding public funds for mental health care, even when a window of opportunity opened under the Carter adminis- tration in the late 1970s. Debilitated and divided, public employees could do little to resist the shattering cutbacks to mental health subsequently enacted under the Reagan administration.

"The Enemy": AFSCME and the APA

By the 1970s, far more states had extended legal and organizing rights to their employees. With the accrual of those rights, public sector unions had become larger and more influential. Of these workers, an overwhelm- ing number worked in public mental health care services. Nearly one in four members of AFSCME – 250,000 of one million – were employed in mental health facilities (RL PPAD finding aid). In fact, the union's membership was so affected by deinstitutionalization that it made that issue the primary focus of its Public Policy Analysis Department in its newly established Washington, DC headquarters in the early 1970s.[30] The union was clearly now aware that federal developments were as con- sequential for its members as state-level ones.

The new AFSCME department's strategy was two-pronged. First, it would launch a massive public relations campaign to highlight the nega- tive aspects of deinstitutionalization and to respond to criticisms inveighed against hospitals. The union had hired journalist Henry Santiestevan, formerly the editor of the UAW monthly *Solidarity* and a regular public relations consultant to César Chávez and the United Farm Workers, to assist the campaign (SNAC n.d.). Santiestevan's report, "Out of Their Beds and into the Streets," emphasized how deinstitutionalization had resulted in "crime, nursing home scandals, and community protests," calling the process a "shell-game for budget cuts, layoffs, and profiteer- ing" (RL PPAD 1/1). In response to these trends, AFSCME demanded "more money"; and, as a member of the AFSCME Public Affairs office elaborated in a memo to Santiestevan: "More doctors and nurses. More training and better reliance upon para-professional and support staff.

---

[30] Other trade unions, such as the Service Employees International Union mentioned in Chapter 1, would also come to represent public mental health care workers; however, at this important political moment for American deinstitutionalization, AFSCME was their primary representative.

A removal of 'profit' as a factor in care for the mentally indigent" (*sic*, Hamilton 1975 in RL WR 60/2). After decades attempting to gain a political voice, public sector workers could now advocate for more revenues to be channeled toward providing mental health care.

Their managers, primarily represented by the APA, were, however, not keen to support the AFSCME. The APA's public sector membership was dwindling. At state mental hospitals, a quarter of positions for staff psychiatrists remained unfilled (Grob 1991, 253). Private psychiatry, meanwhile, was booming. Between 1968 and 1972, the United States added 26 private psychiatric hospitals, all of them for-profit and owned by the many new private corporations entering the health care market.[31] Spending on private outpatient psychiatry now exceeded seven billion dollars (in contemporary USD; per BLS 2023).[32] The financial basis of these funds came neither from the new federal insurance programs nor from private insurance companies, which lacked a national mandate to cover costly mental health services (Grob 1991, 264). Instead, out-of-pocket payments financed the vast majority of private office practice. A study conducted in the early 1970s found that these offices focused almost exclusively on patients with neurotic conditions from the professional and managerial classes. Blue-collar workers, white-collar (nonmanagerial) workers, and schizophrenic patients were underrepresented among patients. African Americans and Hispanics were "virtually absent" from these offices (Grob 1991, 294). In short, the APA's client base had shifted dramatically away from those of state and county hospitals and community mental health centers.

The political-economic interests of AFSCME and the APA were so poorly aligned that AFSCME even referred to the APA as "the enemy," precisely because of its "private sector tilt" (see Wolf to McGarrah 1979 in RL PPAD 3/2). This is not to say that the union did not attempt to form a coalition with its adversary. In a speech to the APA in Philadelphia in 1970, Jerry Wurf, AFSCME's then president, argued that "hospital management can do more ... to please and benefit the worker, and

---

[31] This number reflects the net growth of all private psychiatric hospitals but was primarily driven by those owned by corporations. Not-for-profit private and individually owned for-profit hospitals in fact decreased at this time. In other words, corporation-owned for-profit hospitals drove a dramatic increase in private inpatient psychiatry (NIMH 1977, table A).

[32] This does not include spending on private psychologists, CMHCs, freestanding health clinics, or other mental health outpatient services largely dependent on private psychiatry. See table 2 in Sharfstein and Clark (1978).

consequently, to change the atmosphere surrounding the patient" (RL WS 1/21, 10). But the APA did not accept Wurf's invitation to collaborate. In the same speech, Wurf himself had acknowledged the glaring inequalities of public mental health work. While physicians had raised fees "at a rate 50 percent faster than the cost of living ... the wages of non-supervisory hospital personnel average[d] less than subsistence level in private, non-profit hospitals." The mental health system "helps nobody but the richly rewarded therapists," he would later add in a 1975 speech (RL WS 1/113, 9). In short, AFSCME – having only just found its political footing – saw that a coalition with managers was far from possible.

When a window of opportunity to change mental health policy opened in the late 1970s, therefore, the welfare workforce was not positioned to take advantage of it. Upon his election to the presidency in 1977, Jimmy Carter set up a new President's Commission on Mental Health, a decision prompted, in part, by First Lady Rosalynn Carter's personal interest in mental health.[33] The commission's composition, however, implicitly favored private psychiatry. Bemoaning the paltry presence of labor representatives, AFSCME noted that "most other Commissioners are management or advocates of deinstitutionalization," that is, opponents of public sector psychiatry (see the 1978 memo in RL PPAD 3/6, 2). "Management," of course, included the APA.[34] To counter the private sector's influence, AFSCME requested that the commission appoint its vice president, Albert Blatz, to the Task Panel on Deinstitutionalization, Rehabilitation, and Long-Term Care (RL PPAD 3/6, 1978 memo, 2). The request, though successful, ultimately did little to advance the union's interests in the sea of competing policy positions. In the commission's final report, the mental hospital chaplain was listed as "Father Albert Blatz, St. Peter State Hospital, St. Peter, Minnesota" (PCMH 1978, 83). No mention was made of his position within AFSCME.

---

[33] Although the First Lady was a personal advocate for mental health, people with mental illness were not formally represented on this commission, either (reflecting a pattern set by the 1955 commission). The closest approximation to a client advocate, the National Alliance on Mental Illness, was not established until two years later, in 1979, and by parents, not patients (reflecting a pattern set by the 1963 CMHC Act).

[34] Some of the commission's psychiatrists had public sector experience, such as the APA's Dr. Mildred Mitchell-Bateman and, behind the scenes, the Acting Director of the Division of Mental Health Service, Dr. Steven Sharfstein. At the same time, the APA's formal priorities remained oriented toward the private sector. Moreover, a private, anonymous foundation (possibly the Institute of Medicine) fronted funding to help hire two psychiatrists from elite, private universities to participate in the commission as well. This support further bolstered the influence of privately oriented psychiatrists on its recommendations (Grob 2005; Grob and Goldman 2006, 73).

Unsurprisingly, this commission's recommendations favored private psychiatry as well. Although its final report acknowledged the importance of public finance for mental health care provision (and even went so far as to support the campaign for national health insurance), its more immediate, more realistic recommendations sought to bolster private care. The report recommended that Medicare benefits, for example, should be amended to cover CMHCs and more acute and short-term hospitalization, as well as to reimburse more outpatient care (all services based largely in the private sector). Moreover, the report said nothing of Medicaid's IMD Exclusion. Instead, it criticized the Medicaid program for covering too much institutional care (including in nursing homes). The report asked that states extend Medicaid to pay for more outpatient mental health services and that they invite private health insurers to do the same. Furthermore, the report encouraged the "phase down and where appropriate closing of ... large State mental hospitals" (PCMH 1978, 29). Little was said about the other factors, outside of the health system, influencing deinstitutionalization. A vague recommendation that the administration "explore the feasibility of creating a new system to meet the costs of chronic mental disability" was the only reference that acknowledged the role of the 1972 Social Security Amendments in deinstitutionalization. Personnel recommendations focused not on protecting and expanding public employment but rather on the need to diversify the workforce and develop new curriculums (PCMH 1978, 34). Taken as a whole, the commission's recommendations would benefit private community mental health services – what AFSCME once disparagingly called "Rosalynn Carter's pet cause" – over any form of publicly provided care for poor patients with mental illnesses.[35]

The 1980 Mental Health Systems Act Subdues Public Mental Health Care and Its Employees

The recommendations of the President's Commission directly influenced the resulting Mental Health Systems Act, passed on October 7, 1980. Though lauded as a landmark bill, the legislation in fact undermined public mental health services and its employees. The bill did extend several

---

[35] Drafted in 1981, an internal AFSCME memo drew parallels between the support of two First Ladies, one Democratic, the other Republican, for the private sector: "Just as Rosalynn Carter's pet cause was private community mental health services, so Nancy Reagan's appears to be private community drug abuse problems" (McGarrah to Wurf, WF WF 28/13).

grants for community mental health centers and other services, but no effort was made to guarantee these funds for the longer term. This unstable fiscal provision reflects the divided positions of managers and workers. During the congressional debates about CMHC funding, the APA and AFSCME developed fundamentally different narratives. "Without being self-serving," APA representative Dr. John McGrath exclaimed, "private practitioners and facilities have, in many instances, been left out of the mainstream of the evolution of community mental health." Legislation, in his view, should "go further to provide adequate incentives to the private sector."[36] Encouraging health insurers to cover private outpatient mental health services to the same degree as other health care services was the APA's preferred remedy. Public sector workers, of course, strongly critiqued the APA's victimization narrative:

Those [patients] who have been denied decent treatment from the private mental health care establishment have been consigned to the public institutions where AFSCME members strive to do the best jobs they can under terribly trying circumstances.[37]

The American Federation of State, County, and Municipal Employees advocated that the legislation provide for the state operation of community mental health centers, as well as for the continued support of longer-term state mental health care facilities.[38] After years of mistrust between these two organizations, it was at these hearings that public workers were left most obviously bereft of support by their supervisors.

No attempt was made, furthermore, to redress the gaps in public mental health care coverage created by the 1965 and 1972 Social Security Amendments. This issue, too, lacked the agreement of managers and

---

[36] *Mental Health Systems Act: Hearings on H.R. 4156 and H.R. 3986, Day 2, Before the Subcommittee on Health and Environment of the Committee on Interstate and Foreign Commerce.* 96th Cong. 225 (1972) (statement of Dr. John J. McGrath, on behalf of the American Psychiatric Association).

[37] *Mental Health Systems Act: Hearings on H.R. 4156 and H.R. 3986, Day 2, Before the Subcommittee on Health and Environment of the Committee on Interstate and Foreign Commerce.* 96th Cong. 143 (1972) (statement of Robert McGarrah, Assistant Director, Public Policy Analysis, American Federation of State, County, and Municipal Employees, AFL-CIO).

[38] *Mental Health Systems Act: Hearings on H.R. 4156 and H.R. 3986, Day 2, Before the Subcommittee on Health and Environment of the Committee on Interstate and Foreign Commerce.* 96th Cong. 90–100, 142–45 (1972) (statements of Anthony Carnevale, Director of Legislation, American Federation of State, County, and Municipal Employees, AFL-CIO and Robert McGarrah, Assistant Director, Public Policy Analysis, American Federation of State, County, and Municipal Employees, AFL-CIO, respectively).

workers. While AFSCME repeatedly campaigned to eliminate Medicaid's IMD Exclusion and expand federal disability benefits to those residing in public institutions, the APA remained vague on these issues. Consider the differences between the testimony of both groups. Dr. McGrath of the APA asked Congress to "provide adequate resources, including major modifications in Medicaid, Medicare and the Social Security Disability Insurance to underwrite the income maintenance as well as the non-discriminatory treatment costs for these individuals," but he was not specific about what those modifications should be. Robert McGarrah of AFSCME, however, explicitly requested that:

The SSI [Social Security Disability Insurance] program must also be changed: There is no justification for prohibiting patients in public institutions with more than 16 residents from receiving these funds, when that money is made available to patients in private facilities, even if hundreds of SSI recipients reside in them; Medicaid must be amended to remove funding inequities that prohibit institutional coverage for persons 21–65.[39]

In comparison, federal disability insurance and Medicaid – two social programs for the poor – received little attention from the APA. Such specificity about policy change was only given to Medicare, which the APA still hoped would cover private services more generously.

Perhaps the clearest indicator of the weakness of the position of the US welfare workforce in the 1980 Act was its forced acknowledgment of the inevitability of redundancy, a reality that will contrast sharply with that of their counterparts in France (discussed in Chapter 5), since they secured their position at the height of economic retrenchment. The American Federation of State, County, and Municipal Employees sought to convince Congress to disburse CMHC grants only to states with which the union had negotiated protections for laid-off hospital workers. To do this, AFSCME turned to another set of elected officials: state governors. Several key members of the National Governors Association, however, opposed such restrictions. After all, the governors had few incentives to support this strategy. Exchanging CMHC funds for employee protections would make those funds more difficult to access, not to mention prolong the state's financial obligations

---

[39] *Mental Health Systems Act: Hearings on H.R. 4156 and H.R. 3986, Day 2, Before the Subcommittee on Health and Environment of the Committee on Interstate and Foreign Commerce.* 96th Cong.146 (1972) (statement of Robert McGarrah, Assistant Director, Public Policy Analysis, American Federation of State, County, and Municipal Employees, AFL-CIO).

to workers it no longer needed. Noting the particularly prominent opposition of Pennsylvania's Republican governor Dick Thornburgh, AFSCME turned to his fellow Pennsylvania Republican, Senator Richard Schweiker, a key member of the Subcommittee on Health, for support. Schweiker had once endorsed the idea that the federal government distribute the CMHC funds via the states (previously the funds went directly to the centers). The tactic was successful. A revised bill required the state-level distribution of the CMHC funds and made their uptake conditional on the negotiation of employment protections.[40]

Negative Feedback Prompts Full-Scale Cutbacks to Mental Health from the 1980s Onward

Whatever optimism there was for the Act because of this change, however, lasted less than a month. The political weakness of the welfare workforce was no match for the results of the November 1980 elections. Not only had the Republicans regained the presidency with the election of Ronald Reagan but their control of the Senate also gave them command over a congressional chamber for the first time since 1953. The success of the Republican Party concluded a decade of partisan realignment and ideological reinvention. The party opened the next decade with a more developed neoliberal strategy for reform. In so doing, it moved swiftly to pass the 1981 Omnibus Budget Reconciliation Act, legislation that dramatically restructured federal spending and reduced support for social programs.[41]

Public mental health care was not spared with this Act's passage. Neither the APA nor AFSCME testified at the 1981 bill's sprawling hearings; and the new legislature fully repealed all the financial provisions of the 1980 Mental Health Systems Act.[42] Congress converted the CMHC appropriations into a flexible block-grant program, financed at levels 75 to 80 percent below those promised by the Mental Health Systems Act. The block grants carried few restrictions and no guidelines (Grob and Goldman 2006, 114–15). State hospital workers lost the protection

---

[40] McGarrah to McEntee in RL WR 33/15; Mental Health Systems Act of 1980, Pub. L. No. 96–398, 94 Stat. 1564, codified at 42 U.S.C. §§ 9401–9523, amended § 210 § 225a § 242a § 300m § 1396b § 2689.

[41] Omnibus Budget Reconciliation Act of 1981, Pub. L. 97–35, 95 Stat. 357.

[42] Because the bill dealt with so many social programs, the APA deferred its representation to the AMA and AFSCME to the AFL-CIO Public Employee department, neither of which spoke much about the bill's specific implications for mental health services. For example, *Budget Reconciliation: Hearings, Before the Committee on Post Office and Civil Service.* 97th Cong. (1981).

guarantees they had fought for in the former bill. Private community mental health services, too, would suffer. Limiting the support for the less than 800 CMHCs in operation (a meager fraction of the intended 2,000) meant the program dwindled over time. As of the 2010 National Mental Health Services Survey (SAMHSA 2014), CMHC block grants fund just a third of psychiatric outpatient facilities in America.

Locked into Negative Feedback Loops

In the following years, AFSCME continued to lobby on behalf of its laid-off members. A new public relations document prepared for the early 1980s, "Patients for Sale," doubled down on the language and policy positions of "Out of Their Beds and into the Streets" (RL WR 22/12). It encouraged union locals to add full-time positions devoted to coping with deinstitutionalization (McGarrah to Wurf in RL WR 22/12, 4). In 1980, the Public Policy Department projected spending nearly $400,000 on materials to train its staff on how to negotiate contracts for deinstitutionalizing hospitals (McGarrah to Cowan in RL WR 22/12, 1; in contemporary USD per BLS 2023). But the union lacked the political allies required to be effective. A strategy document from that year makes no mention of involving the APA in its political activities, and instead notes its struggle to find potential partners: "AFSCME stands alone so far in opposition to irresponsible deinstitutionalization" (McGarrah to Wurf in RL WR 22/12, 4).

The return of the Right also meant the exclusion of labor from federal policy-making. The appointment of one AFL-CIO representative to the 44-member Task Force on Private Sector Initiatives was the only official involvement of the Federation in the Reagan administration (McGarrah to Lucy et al. in RL PPAD 16/19). Evidently, the goals of the Task Force did not favor public sector employment. For this reason, the reduction of public mental health services continued. Over the latter half of the 20th century, the number of state and county mental hospitals dropped by well over a third (from 334 at their 1973 peak to 207 in 2003; see table 2 in Atay et al. 2006). Moreover, the scant availability of positions in the community mental health sector made it difficult to support the transfer of their former workers to non-hospital settings. In contrast, in France, mental health workers would be able to work across the full range of inpatient and outpatient settings of the psychiatric sectors (see Chapter 5).

The APA remained passive about many of the core policy issues affecting public mental health services, such as Medicaid's IMD Exclusion and the training of staff for public services. The Association remained active in issues that supported private practice. For example, when the Reagan administration began to purge young people with disabilities from the disability benefit programs to save costs, the Association convened a working group at the Social Security Administration in 1983 to revise the programs' eligibility criteria. The result was the expansion of benefit categories and the requirement that a psychiatrist or psychologist complete a medical assessment for disability claimants before benefits could be denied.[43] Later, in 1985, the APA and the American Hospital Association collaborated to exclude psychiatric specialty inpatient care from Medicare's new prospective payments. The system paid hospitals an average rate in advance for care according to a system of categories known as the "diagnosis-related groups" (DRGs). Excluding costly psychiatric care from this system helped to protect the revenues of private providers (Grob and Goldman 2006, 141). By the 1990s, the mentally ill accounted for more than a third of disability beneficiaries (Erkulwater 2006, 117). It was not until 1999, furthermore, that Congress modified the DRG regulations and implemented a per diem prospective payment system for inpatient psychiatry (Pub. L. No. 105–13).

Initiatives led by career bureaucrats in the federal government did seek to make a few incremental policy changes in support of public mental health services. Notably, a group of public sector supervisors – state mental health directors – encouraged these changes. These state officials lacked the influence of the APA (which could also claim to represent many of them), but they nonetheless worked with the Department of Health, Education, and Welfare to establish a National Plan for the Chronically Mentally Ill.[44] The plan was ambitious and included numerous specific changes to federal programs (including Medicare, Medicaid, and SSI) that would boost support for public sector care. Since the economic and political climate proved too hostile to implement the plan through legislation, the federal government instead pursued smaller scale projects. One of these was the 1986 Program on Chronic Mental Illness to finance the reorganization of local mental health delivery systems in nine large cities. These grants also permitted mental health authorities to subsidize rents for people with mental illnesses. Homelessness had become a

---

[43] For a discussion of the Association's involvement in this issue, see Grob and Goldman (2006, 123–31).

[44] Founded in 1959, the National Association of State Mental Health Program Directors (NASHPD) lacked the historic influence of the APA. Moreover, the group did not supervise state hospital workers directly. This task was left to hospital superintendents, who comprised the APA's small contingent of public psychiatrists (NASMHPD 2018).

pressing problem for the noninstitutionalized since the Reagan administration also cut funds for public housing support. Baby boomers presenting symptoms of schizophrenia (a condition that develops in young adulthood) were among the most affected. They lacked the medical and employment history necessary to both access and afford chronic psychiatric care in the post-asylum era.[45] However, it was the Robert Wood Johnson Foundation, not government, that funded this $80 million program.[46] Indeed, programs like these illustrate the tenuous state of mental health services in America even until today. Short-term, small-scale programs for the most vulnerable cannot rely on secure, long-term public financing, and thus depend on the goodwill of charitable institutions.

Meanwhile, a more stable source of psychiatric care has emerged in a less desirable location: prisons. In a study published in 1984, Steadman and colleagues found that while the state mental hospital population decreased by 64 percent in the 1970s, the prison population increased by nearly the same amount (65 percent). The finding supported the classic sociological hypothesis that "if the prison services are extensive, the asylum population is relatively small and the reverse also tends to be true" (Penrose 1939). However, the authors of the study, like many others who have examined the expansion of the American carceral system, underscored that the relationship was not quite so simple in the United States. Many of the factors that spurred mass incarceration had little to do with those that deinstitutionalized the mentally ill (e.g., the reliance of victims' movements on law-and-order politicians in absence of a supportive welfare state, the criminalization of drug activity, and the lucrative development of the private prison industry).[47] But the connection remains. As Parsons explores, the same conservative politicians who reduced funds for welfare and medical services also paid more attention to security and punishment. Those who had been involuntarily confined in mental hospitals were now often involuntarily confined in prisons instead (Parsons 2018). Causes aside, the result was that many people with mental illnesses found themselves living

---

[45] Although much of the public perceives a connection between President Reagan, the deinstitutionalized, and homelessness, it is important to underscore that Reagan played a more direct role in cutting housing support than he did in cutting funds from state mental hospitals – which, as shown, had begun to depopulate decades prior. Moreover, not all of the homeless population suffered from chronic mental illness; many had simply suffered from the housing cuts. For a theoretical discussion on the popular association between these factors, see Mossman (1997).

[46] In contemporary USD (per BLS 2023).

[47] For a discussion of the lessons of psychiatric deinstitutionalization for penal reform, see Gottschalk (2012).

in prisons, which in turn became providers of mental health care (Fuller Torrey et al. 2012). Some of the largest psychiatric institutions are in fact prisons (Ford 2015). As Lara-Millán (2021) has shown, the US prison system is poorly equipped to support people with mental illness, aggravating the inadequacies of the medical system in this area.

Although the Reagan (and then George H. W. Bush) era was followed by a period of Democratic governance, the Clinton administration adopted a Third Way approach to social spending (as did many of its peer governments in other countries). The economic retrenchment of the 1996 welfare reforms exemplifies how Democrats continued many of the policies inherited from the Reagan era. A small window of opportunity emerged for public psychiatric workers (and patients) during the attempts to enact a universal health program in the early 1990s, but this proved too costly for insurers, and too unattractive to private practitioners, to succeed in Congress. The return of the Right in the early 2000s continued to favor maintaining the status quo. It was not until the enactment of the Affordable Care Act in 2010 under President Obama that some attention was paid to financing mental health services, and even so, the bill's mental health reforms were limited, as noted in the discussion of the American mental health system in Chapter 2. Moreover, the core challenge of financing mental health reforms endures. To date, the CMHC program hardly exists, insurers have limited incentive to cover psychiatric care, and Medicaid excludes "institutions for mental disease" from its benefit package.

ALTERNATIVE EXPLANATIONS

In the preceding pages, I have argued that the absence of a coalition between public sector workers (represented primarily by AFSCME) and managers (represented primarily by private practitioners in the APA) produced negative policy feedback loops that gradually reduced the supply of mental health care services and the overall strength of its workforce. Although the next chapter will demonstrate how the presence of such a coalition produced the opposite result in France, here I consider three main alternative explanations for the American outcome.

First, I explore whether and how pro-deinstitutionalization social movements played an outsized role in reducing services in the United States. Second, I address the role of American federalism in producing these outcomes. Third, I consider whether postwar development of the American welfare state – which became increasingly racialized, restricted, and privatized as a whole – influenced the trajectory of mental health policy. Each of these explanations helps to fill out the picture of deinstitutionalization in the postwar period, but none offers a sufficient account of its core policy drivers.

Alternative Explanation 1: The Pro-deinstitutionalization Movement

There is no question that the public support for deinstitutionalization gained political momentum in the United States. Some might even go so far as to call it a social movement.[48] Its development, however, was more a symptom than a cause of underfunded public mental health care. In the words of a leading AFSCME lobbyist, "virtually every patient's rights lawsuit in this country can be traced directly to overcrowding, understaffing, and inadequate funding of state institutions" (McGarrah to McKinney in RL WR 28/14, 10). Hollywood, the press, and the academic community rightly drew attention to the often inhumane and scandalous conditions of the decrepit state and county mental hospitals. Public outcry rightly followed. Rather than support the expansion of public funds, however, these complaints unconsciously aligned with the interests of private psychiatrists. As Dunst (in Kritsotaki et al. 2016) has also argued, these movements both arose from and contributed to the pattern of deinstitutionalization in America.

Consider the example of academic social criticism. A number of social scientists, both in the United States and abroad, had begun to question the dominance of the psychiatric profession as arbiters of social norms. The publications of scholars such as Thomas Szasz (e.g., *The Myth of Mental Illness*, 1961, and *The Manufacture of Madness*, 1970) and Erving Goffman (most notably, *Asylums*, 1961) circulated among readers who were sympathetic to similar liberationist ideas in Black, feminist, and other critical thought. Many of them responded by rejecting state-operated psychiatric services, believing that the termination of these services would result in the termination of psychiatric oppression, too. When this academic conversation was taken up by the public, however, it had the unintended consequence of bolstering arguments for privatizing services. For example, many private clinical psychologists espoused a milder form

---

[48] Although deinstitutionalization is frequently referred to as a "social movement," that appellation may be a misnomer. A standard definition offered by Tarrow (1994), for example, distinguishes the collective, sustained, and highly participatory qualities of social movements from the more independent work of an advocacy group or mere public discontent. It is not clear that the support for deinstitutionalization described here would meet these criteria.

of this anti-psychiatric critique by arguing against the medical model of mental illness. Given the difference between their clients and those of the public mental hospitals, their therapeutic services were sustainable with less public funding. Drawing on these arguments to advocate for licensing and certification equivalence, the profession became more popular and its size nearly doubled in the 1980s (Grob and Goldman 2006, 47).

A similar pattern followed in the courts. Building on critical legal scholarship that equated involuntary commitment to a mental hospital with incarceration in a prison without due process (Birnbaum 1960), advocates began to pursue legal recourse for patients mistreated by state psychiatry in the 1960s.[49] A subsequent ripple of court decisions in the early 1970s made it more difficult for states to treat patients against their will.[50] But by chipping away at government authority in the area of mental illness, these decisions inadvertently facilitated the ongoing financial retrenchment of its services. Reducing treatment became easier than imposing it.

Politically, welfare workers were too weak to reverse these trends. Delayed mobilization by AFSCME affected its potency in the courts as much as it did in Congress. In a 1973 internal memo, nearly two full years after the first court ruling in 1971, an analyst raised the point that:

AFSCME has not utilized the full potential of the court decision ... it would seem that *Wyatt v Stickney* could be used by us in numerous cases to demand adequate staff and facilities both for the patients and for the employees. It could also become an important factor in the whole problem of closing down institutions. (Miller to Hein in RL PPAD 3/20)

Although the memo included a host of research on how to reframe the ruling as an advocacy tool for significant service expansion, that same year the Supreme Court was already ruling that involuntary commitment was illegal in all cases of "non-dangerous" individuals. Those "capable of surviving safely in freedom" should do so.[51] This decision made it even more difficult for AFSCME to advocate for service expansions. Moreover, the financial means available to support AFSCME's surmised

---

[49] In the United States, interest groups often turn to the courts in the absence of alternative routes to political influence (e.g., through labor and welfare institutions, through Congress and political parties). As a result, though, mobilization in the courts can foreclose other opportunities to redress concerns elsewhere. For an example, see Gottschalk (2006).

[50] Wyatt v. Stickney 325 F. Supp. 781 (United States District Court, M. D. Alabama March 12, 1971); Lessard v. Schmidt, 413 F. Supp. 1318 (United States District Court, E. D. Wisconsin May 28, 1976); O'Connor v. Donaldson, 422 US 563 (United States Supreme Court June 26, 1976); see also Gillon (2000, 106).

[51] O'Connor v. Donaldson, 422 US 563 (United States Supreme Court June 26, 1976).

strategy had dropped precipitously in the intervening years. Rather than raise revenues to provide adequate staff and resources, by that point states were more likely to respond to inadequacies by shutting down institutions in their entirety.[52]

Alternative Explanation 2: American Federalism

Scholars of American social policy often point to the role of the country's fraught federal–state relations as a factor driving its fragmentation (Lieberman 1998; Mettler 1998; Michener 2018).[53] Public mental health services, too, encountered this challenge. The lack of coordination between, on the one hand, federal-level CMHC grants, Medicare, Medicaid, nursing home grants, and disability insurance and, on the other hand, state-level hospital financing contributed to America's mishandling of deinstitutionalization. Complicating matters further was that the state-level policies also varied. This variation affected not only when, where, and to what extent public employees could unionize but also what their mental health policy agenda might be. In fact, for most of the 1970s, AFSCME lacked a unified policy position on deinstitutionalization. "As I understand it," the author of a 1979 internal memo worked out, "we [AFSCME] are totally against it [deinstitutionalization] in Pennsylvania, with a modified acceptance in New York State, [and] in Milwaukee we are both against and for" (Dowling to Wurf in RL

---

[52] The APA, for its part, was also concerned with some of these campaigns – especially that of civil liberties – though for other reasons. Like its counterparts in other countries, the American psychiatric profession sought to maintain control over medical decision-making. For example, the APA's primary agenda item during the debates over the 1980 Mental Health Systems Act was to defeat the effort to enact a patient's bill of rights (Grob and Goldman 2006, 110–12). The APA disagreed with civil liberties activists and many legal scholars that legislating patient protections would improve care. And at this effort, they were successful. The 1980 Act deleted virtually all mandates regarding patient protections, a policy outcome that the 1981 Omnibus Bill also left untouched. Still, the overarching legal framework that guides patient rights in American psychiatry remained quite permissive, as per the court rulings of the early 1970s.

[53] The checks and balances across the other US political institutions, ranging from the Supreme Court's power of judicial review to the president's power to veto congressional legislation, can make it difficult to pass cohesive and generous social policy as well. I have discussed the role of the courts in the previous section. Since the historical period studied in this chapter saw few instances of divided government (in fact none for most of it, from 1958 to 1981) and more party discipline than the present, the executive and legislative branches generally did not exercise their veto points in mental health policy-making. This section therefore focuses on American federalism as the remaining major institutional challenge.

PPAD 34/4). How could the welfare workforce fully respond to budget cuts with so little federal–state coordination and so much cross-state variation?

Although the following chapter will discuss how French workers in fact used policy decentralization precisely to promote their interests, several developments in the American case also question the extent to which federalism is solely to blame for its mental health care outcomes. First, the cross-state variation in mental health policy in effect underscores the critical role of public labor–management coalitions. That workers could not form this alliance with their supervisors at the federal level does not mean that they could not do so at the state level. Note that the vast majority of public mental health care employees were local, not federal, employees, so they first sought redress from state governments (and governors, as the third feedback cycle showed). Indeed, the presence or absence of that coalition at the state level often contributed to the local variation in public mental health financing and services.[54] Coalition formation at the state level nonetheless became more complicated as federal and private health services and benefits developed, for they offered managers more opportunities to exit public employment and enter private practice.[55]

At this point, and second, AFSCME took on a robust coordinating role between the federal and state levels. Consider its actions during the passing of the 1980 Mental Health Systems Act. Turning to an alternative set of public supervisors, state governors, the workers managed to rewrite the terms of the federal bill: States would receive CMHC funds only if they negotiated employment protections for state hospital workers. Although workers were not able to develop this coordination until it was too late in the deinstitutionalization process, they nonetheless demonstrated a capacity to supersede the challenges of federalism to promote their economic interests and procure revenues.

---

[54] State workforce laws and management policies also vary substantially, such that some public mental health care employees likely enjoyed more benefits than others. Workers in some states might have been able to draw on some resources more than their counterparts in other states (or even in the federal government, which has been known to cap employee numbers in the past). Even the prestige attributed to state work can vary. These resources could have further empowered coalitions in some states and helped them achieve their local aims.

[55] Here is an example of how institutions can challenge alliance possibilities, as noted in Chapter 1. Although American federalism did not irrevocably alter actors' behavior, it posed another obstacle to forming a public labor–management coalition (whose impact on policy outcomes is more direct).

Alternative Explanation 3: The Effect of Race
on the American Welfare State

As in other countries, the welfare state expanded in the United States after the Second World War. Unlike other countries, however, it also developed its more racialized, limited, as well as privatized character. The distribution of US social benefits often falls along racial lines, with limited public social provision for low-income, non-whites and more generous, if privatized, social provision for whites employed both formally and stably. Did this pattern of distribution also shape the mental health care outcomes? Limited research has examined this question. A possible answer proceeds in two parts:

To begin, it appears that this logic could not initiate the decline of public mental services in the early part of the postwar period. In the 1950s, 1960s, and 1970s, the population of institutionalized patients was primarily elderly and white.[56] This group was broadly perceived as "deserving" of social support, indeed this presumption was an important driver of the 1965 Social Security Amendments, which redistributed generously to that group. Perhaps perceptions would have been different had the patient populations of state and county mental hospitals been primarily non-white and working age, two factors (race and ability to work) that can code benefit recipients as "undeserving." But this was not the case. Rather, as illustrated, the APA and AFSCME seemed more concerned with the distributive implications by patient diagnosis, which largely shaped their ability to pay for their own care. As private services for the milder conditions of the YAVIS population grew, public services for indigent patients with chronic and severe mental illness, such as schizophrenia, declined. In keeping with the theoretical expectations laid out in Chapter 1, only public sector employees advocated on behalf of the most disenfranchised.

By the late 20th century, however, several developments combined that may have shifted the perceived target population of mental health policy away from elderly white women and toward unemployed, homeless, even "violent" Black men. First, the Great Migration of African Americans from the American South to northern cities rendered them a more visible, urbanized population in the eye of the public in the 1960s.[57]

---

[56] A government report exploring these trends attributed them to numerous factors, including the expanding elderly population and the "racist and discriminatory practices" that redirected some patients to correctional facilities instead of medical care (Kramer 1977).

[57] Jonathan Metzl (2009) has argued that, because this visibility coincided with the political unrest of the civil rights movement, it contributed to the gradual evolution in schizophrenia's diagnostic criteria. Metzl demonstrated that psychiatrists began to adapt the criteria to justify the institutionalization of protestors; schizophrenia was becoming a "Black disease."

When deindustrialization then displaced many of these (mostly male) Black workers from their northern industrial jobs in the late 1970s, it left them highly dependent on means-tested social welfare programs. That these benefits experienced the sharp social welfare cuts of the 1980s and early 1990s only exacerbated Black urban poverty and, in many cases, homelessness. The comingling of this population with those recently deinstitutionalized on the streets and in halfway houses (all of whom were also targets of the racially coded "war on drugs") ultimately produced the image of "psychiatric ghetto" in the public's mind (Gillon 2000, 104; Grob 1991, 261). This characterization, both unfair and untrue, nonetheless may have shifted public presumptions about the mentally ill, undermining the perceived deservingness of expanded public mental health services over time. Consider the emergence of "NIMBY" – Not In My Back Yard – campaigns in the late 20th century. Public outcry over the psychiatric ghetto tended to rally around making it less visible, not delivering the medical, housing, and employment services necessary to address its root causes.

If race shaped mental health care, then, it did so in ways different from conventional expectations. While the target population of many other areas of US social policy (e.g., cash assistance) is consistently perceived as Black and undeserving, that is not the case in mental health care, where the target population was initially perceived as white. It is difficult, then, to attribute the postwar launch of negative supply-side policy feedback to systematic or interpersonal racism. Rather, this explanation may have become a complementary one over subsequent feedback cycles. Absent a robust coalition of welfare workers in this area, changing perceptions about who constituted its target population rendered these services even less worthy of public funds.

In conclusion, explanations for the pattern of American deinstitutionalization and the precipitous decline of public mental health services cannot stand without giving substantial attention to the limited strength of public sector trade unions and their unsympathetic supervisors during the postwar period. The importance of this unformed alliance will become even more clear in the next chapter: In sharp contrast to the American case, a powerful alliance of workers and managers in French mental health care pivoted the pattern of deinstitutionalization in the opposite direction. The deinstitutionalization of mental asylums did not decrease mental health services; in fact, it increased them. Three cycles of positive supply-side policy feedback, prompted by an alliance between workers and managers, contributed to this outcome.

TABLE 4.1 *Within-case process-tracing tests, United States*

Empirical questions (and type of process-tracing test, Van Evera 1997; Bennett 2010)	Evidence	Interpretation
Core theoretical argument 1: Public sector workers and managers do not express the same preferences for public service expansion.		
1.A. Do workers mobilize in favor of public service maintenance and expansion? (Hoop test)	Statement from AFSCME headquarters during the first feedback cycle; and later, political lobbying efforts of the AFSCME Public Policy Analysis Department.	Yes, public mental health workers expressed a preference for, and then mobilized in favor of, maintaining and expanding public psychiatric services.
1.B. Does the organization representing public psychiatric managers prevent them from expressing a preference for public service maintenance and expansion? (Hoop test)	Results of the 1955 Joint Commission; APA statements during the 1960 Great Society reforms and the 1980 Mental Health Act.	Yes, the joint organization of public psychiatric managers with private practitioners prevented the former from expressing an independent and singular preference for public service maintenance and expansion.
1.C. Do workers and managers fail to form a coalition? (Hoop test)	No coalition in the first or second feedback cycles; outright identification of APA as "the enemy" by AFSCME in the third.	Yes, public sector workers and managers failed to form a coalition during deinstitutionalization.
Core theoretical argument 2: Without a coalition of public sector managers and workers, policy-makers do not accede to public service expansion; thus the following causal mechanisms are absent:		
2.A. Brokerage: Do public managers fail to use the privileged tools at their disposal to secure and expand the delivery of public services? (Smoking-gun test)	APA trades its silence on CMHC staffing grants for the political support of AMA during the first feedback cycle.	At the national level, public psychiatric managers did not broker demands of workers during deinstitutionalization.

2.B. Adaptive expectations: Do policy-makers avoid concessions without fear of retribution from the coalition? (Smoking-gun test)	Tenuous congressional support for CMHC appropriation in the first feedback cycle; statement by Senator Russell Long in the second feedback cycle; disagreements of state governors over redundancy protections in the third feedback cycle.	Policy-makers do not appear to have feared retribution from the welfare workforce for cutbacks.

Core theoretical argument 3: Negative feedback undermines the welfare workforce, relaunching the feedback cycle.

3.A. Does the public sector workforce decrease as funds for public services decrease? (Hoop test)	After the 1960s, private psychiatric services and spending increase, CMHCs depend more on private funds, and public mental hospitals decrease.	Trends in the distribution of service provision suggests that the size of the public sector psychiatric workforce decreased over time.
3.B. Do workforce mobilizations become weaker as funds expand? (Hoop test)	AFSCME pivots its attention to protections for redundancies in the third feedback cycle.	The mobilization of public sector psychiatric workers became less ambitious as deinstitutionalization progressed.

Alternative explanations:

Alt.A. The decline of US public mental health services is the inevitable result of the pro-deinstitutionalization movement.	1973 AFSCME memo about legal strategy. (Passes a doubly-decisive test standard)	The pro-deinstitutionalization movement was partly the result of the political weakness of the welfare workforce.
Alt.B. The decline of US public mental health services is the inevitable result of the federal system.	Workers can and do seek redress from state governors; and AFSCME plays a coordinating role across the federal system. (Passes a hoop test standard)	The US federal system does not appear to have overdetermined the failure of the labor–management coalition in this policy area.
Alt.C. The decline of US public mental health services is the inevitable result of the racialized welfare system.	In the postwar period, patients in public mental hospitals were primarily elderly and white; later, several policy developments combined that may have shifted public perceptions about mental health care's target population. (Passes a hoop test standard)	It is difficult to attribute the initial decline in public mental health care to racial animus against its clients, though this explanation may have become a complementary one over subsequent feedback cycles.

5

Deinstitutionalization in France

At the end of the Second World War, France's prospects for expanding mental health care were similar to those of the United States, if, perhaps, a little dimmer. The war had devastated the mental health system under the Vichy regime: Between 40,000 and 45,000 psychiatric patients died of famine, which nearly halved the population living in asylums (from about 100,000 before the war). Although the population residing in psychiatric institutions rose over the next few years, very little political and policy attention was paid to the ailing system. Hospitals were at the brink of closure (Bouhallier 2021). By the time American legislators were making an explicit congressional commitment to expanding the public mental health outpatient system in 1963, French policy-makers had only developed a loose set of suggestions for local officials to consider in a 1960 administrative circular.

Yet this initially insignificant administrative circular has more recently gained mythical status as the founding text of one of the world's largest public mental health systems (see Figure 1.1). The document was the first to formally propose the concept of "sectorization," in which the state would supply diverse care services across geographically delimited catchment areas (each of them a "sector"). Although the concept was not immediately implemented, it eventually became the cornerstone of the "French way" of deinstitutionalizing the mentally ill in the second half of the 20th century (Demay and Demay 1982). This alternative approach, however, has received little attention from international analysts. In this chapter, I offer an English-language discussion of the political-economic development of the French case, finding that the mobilization of workers against deinstitutionalization pressures induced policy-makers to instead expand mental health services.

As I theorize in Chapter 1, a coalition of public mental health workers and their managers was crucial to this expansion of services. An independent and unified organization of the public psychiatrists who supervised hospital personnel – the Trade Union of Psychiatric Hospital Physicians (Syndicat des médecins des hôpitaux psychiatriques; that is, the Syndicat) – served as a critical conduit for public workers' petitions.[1] But that coalition did not form until well after the administrative circular was published. As in the previous chapter, I trace three supply-side policy feedback cycles. Figures 5.1–5.3 illustrate each cycle in turn, and Table 5.2 at the end of this chapter formalizes how the evidence meets methodological expectations.

THE FIRST FEEDBACK LOOP: THE LIMITED DEVELOPMENT OF MENTAL HEALTH SECTORS

Most observers trace the origins of psychiatric sectorization in France to an administrative circular issued in 1960. For confirmation, look no further than the title of a recent 469-page government evaluation report: "Organization and Functioning of Psychiatric Care Resources, 60 Years after the Circular of March 15, 1960" (Lopez and Turan-Pelletier 2017). But the circular, though intellectually significant for its novel proposals, was hardly landmark legislation. Nonetheless, any analysis of the French approach to deinstitutionalization, and its consequently extensive system of state-funded outpatient and inpatient psychiatric care, must begin with this "revolutionary" text (Bauduret 2002). While its authority may be exaggerated, indeed mythical, the circular marks the first time that public managers successfully persuaded government authorities to allocate new funds to the mental health sector in the postwar period. Its

---

[1] In the language of postwar French health policy, the Syndicat's members were often "*médecins-chefs*" or "*chefs de service*" (and later, "*chefs de secteur*"), a role likened to the "boss" of a "medical fiefdom" (de Pouvourville 1986, 408; Gay 2011, 19; and discussed in personal communication). In general, these physicians could influence the scale and distribution of the health care workforce by requesting additional staff for their specialty area through a national recruitment system. In psychiatric establishments, furthermore, their managerial responsibilities and authority increased, as *médecins-chefs* directed entire hospitals (and sectors). Although nonmedical hospital directors began to emerge in general health care in this period, *médecins-chefs* in psychiatry carried on the roles described in Chapter 3 and retained substantial control over staff through the 1980s (Ayme 1995, 407; Mossé and Tchobanian 1999, 149). This chapter, then, continues to follow the Syndicat as the primary representative of public psychiatric managers as deinstitutionalization unfolded.

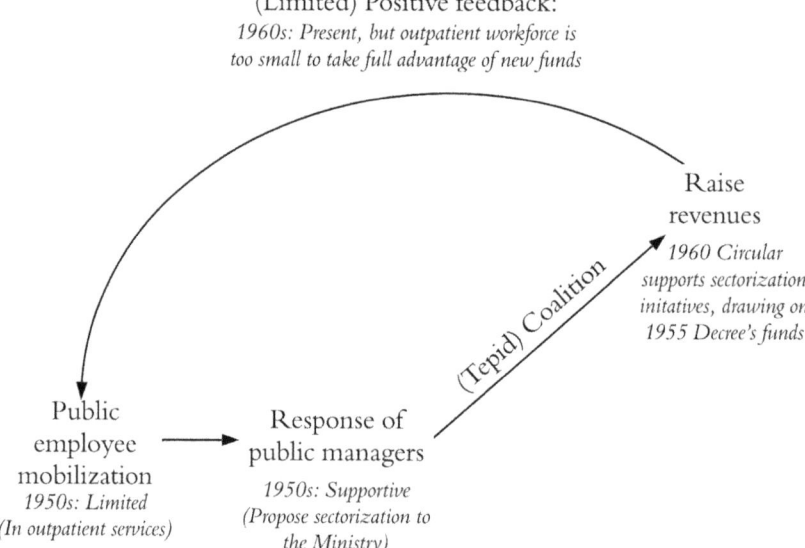

FIGURE 5.1 First supply-side policy feedback loop, postwar French mental health care

full implementation, however, was delayed. As this first (stunted) feedback loop will show, the absence of a coalition between public managers and workers slowed the take-up of funds in outpatient services (see Figure 5.1). Without a robust mental health workforce advocating for more resources for the mental health sector, a generous set of financial supports were left unused for more than a decade.

Public Managers without Public Workers: The Tepid Origins of Sectorization

At the close of the Second World War, both public psychiatric managers and workers had the legal right to organize. Represented by the Syndicat, managers had begun to develop an independent political voice on matters of mental health policy. The Communist-affiliated General Confederation of Labor (Confédération générale du travail, or CGT) and its more independent offshoot, Workers' Force (Force ouvrière, hereafter FO), had begun to organize workers in mental hospitals as well (Bouhallier 2021). But because outpatient services were limited at this time, worker organization remained more limited in that setting, too. As a result, a formal coalition between managers and workers on outpatient public mental health services had not yet formed, and this weakened the overall support for expanding and rebuilding psychiatric care after the war.

The relative novelty of the Syndicat, which had only just formed in 1946, also weakened the organization on several fronts. By the late 1940s, a rival group – the Trade Union of Nervous System Psychiatrists (Syndicat des médecins français spécialistes du système nerveux) – had formed to represent private practitioners and neurologists. Moreover, its members voted to affiliate with the Confederation of French Medical Trade Unions (Confédération des syndicats médicaux français, or CSMF), France's powerful medical association that also favored private practice. These private practitioners jockeyed for attention from the Ministry of Health and Social Affairs (hereafter the Ministry), which in turn offered them spots on its advisory councils. In 1949, the Ministry even appointed the founder of the Trade Union of Nervous System Psychiatrists, Dr. Georges Heuyer, as the president of the reformed "Commission on Mental Health" (hereafter the Commission), a consultation body that had until then been reserved for public psychiatrists ("Séance du 24 mai 1949" in AN 19950173/1, 2). In the words of one prominent public psychiatrist, Dr. Georges Daumezon, the move rendered relations between his Syndicat and the Ministry "practically broken" (cited in Ayme 1995, 41).

The Administrative Circular of 1960 Makes Funds Available, If Indirectly, for New Mental Health "Sectors"

Nearly a decade passed without much policy change in public mental health until a personnel change at the Ministry opened a window of opportunity for the Syndicat. A group of bureaucrats sympathetic to the expansion of public mental health services appointed one of its leading members, Dr. Hubert Mignot, as "Technical Counselor" to the Ministry's Bureau of Psychiatry. Dr. Mignot used the opportunity to promote the Syndicat's vision for mental health reform, a concept called "sectorization" that had first appeared in a memo released by the Syndicat in 1947 (Ayme 1995, 51–52; Henckes 2007, 786). Over the following years, the proposals in this 1947 memo had filtered into the Ministry through reports written by members of the Syndicat sitting on the Commission.[2]

---

[2] See, for example, Lauzier and Godeau 1948 in AN 19950173/1. Note that the Ministry expressed serious reservations about this proposition at the time, such that its authorization of the sectors would have been unlikely without the Syndicat's advocacy for them ("Section technique: Séance du 19 octobre 1948," in AN 19950173/1).

The Commission's 1955 report on psychiatric hospitals, for example, is particularly illustrative. In the report, the authors advocated for the expansion of government-financed mental health care services (especially outpatient services).[3] They argued that this expansion would equitably distribute mental health services across the territory, a policy frame that Lynch (2020) has shown to be especially potent in France. Drawing on these ideas, the bureaucrats of the Ministry's Bureau of Psychiatry drafted an administrative circular with suggestions for local officials on how to develop their public mental health system. Local authorities were to take stock of their psychiatric resources and design a program in line with the Ministry's new mental health policy vision set out in the circular. With the intention of "separating the patient from his family and his environment as little as possible," a team of mental health professionals would care for the needs of a catchment area of about 67,000 persons.[4] Each of the French *départements* (subnational units) would constitute an overarching "sector," which would coordinate these teams and their catchment areas ("subsectors," *sous-secteurs*).[5] It would be up to the chief psychiatrist for each sector, in conjunction with the director of the local health office, to determine the specific arrangement of services, in accordance, the Ministry presupposed, with population needs (1960 circular, 9). Those *départements* that lacked a chief psychiatrist (a not infrequent occurrence) would assign that task to another official, namely the *département*'s health director.

The 1960 administrative circular recommended, but did not require, that each sector include several types of services. Although expanding hospital capacity was at the top of the list (French officials were painfully embarrassed that the supply of beds in their country lagged far behind the World Health Organization standard at the time),[6] the authors of the French circular also recommended establishing services in each sector that resembled

---

[3] The 1955 "Rapport sur l'équipement psychiatrique, d'un territoire dépourvu de toute formation spécialisée" was discussed at multiple meetings, for example, December 19, 1955; February 28, 1956; October 27, 1959; October 27, 1959; and November 29, 1959 (AN 19950173/1).

[4] Circulaire du 15 mars 1960 relative au programme d'organisation et d'équipement des départements en matière de lutte contre les maladies mentales. Ministère de la santé publique et de la population, Direction générale de la santé publique (7e bureau), 2–3; hereafter "1960 circular."

[5] I simply will use the term "sector" to refer to subsectors from now on, as policy-makers and professionals began to do over the following decades.

[6] France had 2.1 compared to the WHO-recommended 3 beds per 1,000 population (1960 circular, 6; Ayme 1995, 261).

those promoted by their American counterparts advocating community mental health: an outpatient mental hygiene center, preferably integrated into a community center that served other social needs (*centre polyvalent*); a day hospital (a service directly inspired by the United States and other countries); a rehabilitation center; and a protected employment workshop.

Moreover, the circular remained agnostic as to whether these services should be public or private, perhaps a response to the protests of private and academic neuropsychiatrists, who disliked its approach.[7] In fact, the circular implied that nonprofit organizations would jump at the opportunity to enter this newly created market: "Day hospitals, re-habilitation centers, protected employment workshops are projects that above all will interest private, not-for-profit organizations, acting in conjunction with mental hygiene physicians at psychiatric hospitals." Nonetheless, the circular continued, "nothing prevents interested local public authorities from pursuing such projects themselves" (1960 circular, 8). Moreover, the circular envisioned the sector as a sort of private–public partnership, whereby private clinical psychiatrists and neuropsychiatrists based in universities could "harmonize" their services with public and not-for-profit actors (11–12).

How did this simple, unbinding document jump-start the first feedback loop and eventually gain mythical status as the founding document of contemporary French mental health policy? Part of the answer lies in its obscure funding source. To support the implementation of its proposals, especially the non-hospital services, the Ministry suggested that actors draw on the public monies made available by the Decree of May 20, 1955 (1960 circular, 1). This earlier document expanded the availability of central government funds for mental hygiene dispensaries from a mere 20 percent to a whopping 80 percent of operational costs, extending the mandate of another policy produced in 1954.[8] Following the enactment

---

[7] See, for example, the debate between Drs. Heuyer, representing the private and academic psychiatrists, and Bonnafé, representing public psychiatrists, in the "Procès-verbal de la séance du 29 novembre 1955" (AN 19950173/1, 3; also Henckes 2011a, 172). Note that not all in the *Syndicat* immediately supported the sectorization policy. An article written in the early 1960s in *l'Information psychiatrique* "Contre le secteur," attests this reality. However, by the mid 1960s, more than 80 percent of the attendees at an affiliated scientific conference (*les Journées nationales de l'Évolution psychiatrique*, 1965–67) approved a White Paper adopting the sectorization policy (Leguay 2002).

[8] Décret 55-571 du 20 mai 1955 sur la prophylaxie des maladies mentales, pris dans le cadre des pouvoirs spéciaux accordés au Gouvernement par la loi du 2 avril 1955, *Journal officiel de la République française*, 5068–69; Loi 54-439 du 15 avril 1954 sur le traitement des alcooliques dangereux pour autrui, *Journal officiel de la République française*, 3827–29.

of a law targeting the treatment of alcoholism, the Ministry had developed the dispensary program to tend to the unwelcome disruptions of various "social ills" (*fléaux sociaux*). Indeed, much of the Ministry's initial attention given to mental health was motivated by the special case of alcoholism, but it soon expanded the definition of "social ills" to encompass many other conditions treated in psychiatric hospitals, such as psychosis.[9] Several addendum documents also released in 1955 made it clear that the funds could serve multiple purposes.[10]

Limited Feedback and the "Long Sleep" of French Mental Health Services

Yet the funds allocated by the 1955 decree – though generous and relatively unconstrained during the booming *Trente Glorieuses* (1945–75) – would not be tapped to implement the 1960 circular for over a decade. Indeed, few sectors were established in the 1960s (Benamouzig 2005, 103; Coffin 2005, 238). A needs assessment produced in the following decade noted that fewer than half of the anticipated sectors and their associated administrative infrastructure had been developed.[11] Some analysts have even referred to this period as the "long sleep" of French mental health services (Murard and Fourquet 1975, 195). Looking back on this period, the policy-maker Jean-François Bauduret lamented that "public psychiatry has lost [more than a decade] and has passed up a historic opportunity to rapidly reform itself thanks to a favorable economic context and a flexible and effective financial mechanism" (Bauduret 2002, 2).

The political dynamics of the first feedback loop explain this delay. Although public managers conceptualized sectorization and secured

---

[9] For documentation of the Ministry's interest in alcoholism, see the records of the Commission des maladies mentales (Archives Nationales) from the early 1960s.

[10] Décret 55-687 du 21 mai 1955 portant règlement d'administration publique pour la détérmination de la part des départements et des communes dans les dépenses d'aide sociale, *Journal officiel de la République française*, 5219–20, Annexe; Circulaire 133 du 4 octobre 1955, Application du Décret 55-571 du 20 mai 1955 Dispensaires d'hygiène mentale (Direction de l'hygiène sociale, 2e Bureau), *Bulletin du Ministère de la santé publique et de la population*, 1955, 395–96.

[11] A letter from the Ministry, dated 1975, claims that only 371 sectors had signed agreements to confirm their status (*conventions de secteur*), of the 737 planned sectors. Moreover, not all sectors had a chief psychiatrist (only 607, according to the letter), only 93 had complied with the expected departmental commitments (*règlements départementaux de lutte contre les maladies mentales, l'alcoolisme, and les toxicomanies*), and only 73 had established the requisite mental health councils (see Mamelet letter in AN 19910084/30/Documents de travail/Sectorisation).

some financial resources for it, the public mental health workforce in non-hospital services remained too small in the 1960s to exert significant pressure on government to increase expenditures on the sectors. Note that hospital workers did mobilize to protect their employment in the period immediately following the Second World War. Bouhallier (2021), for example, shows how the CGT and FO unions representing employees of psychiatric hospitals in the Seine *département* resisted closures by setting up "defense committees." Moreover, he finds that the support of public psychiatrists for the unions' efforts "undoubtedly influenced" policy-makers, who ultimately conceded. But, for the most part, hospital workers in this period were demanding support from more established funding streams, such as Social Security (see Table 5.1). Employment in the non-hospital sectorized services remained too small to generate robust demand for funds in those alternative settings. It was not until the second feedback loop that the number of workers in outpatient services grew, putting pressure on managers and the Ministry to use the funds made available in 1955 and expand the sectors as suggested by the 1960 circular.

Until then, the 1960 circular remained a marginal document. Many reformers would have preferred a more substantial commitment to public psychiatry from government, perhaps made via order, decree, or even legislation. Instead, they received an unpublished set of guidelines, with some suggested, but undelivered, funds from the 1955 decree. Those funds would prove to be crucial to the expansion of public mental health services. In some ways, the (unintended) founding document of French sectorization is not the Circular of May 15, 1960, but the Decree of May 20, 1955, because of its attached funding resources. Nevertheless, over the following decade neither document was of immediate consequence.

THE SECOND FEEDBACK LOOP: THE EXPANSION OF THE MENTAL HEALTH SECTORS

It was not until the student and labor protests of May 1968 that the situation changed for the politics of mental health care in France. The student and labor activism of that political moment motivated the Syndicat to participate in solidarity movements. When public managers launched an extended administrative strike at the peak of the 1968 protests, government leaders made several concessions that would expand the pipeline of public mental health workers in both inpatient and outpatient settings and augment the administrative and political levers available to public

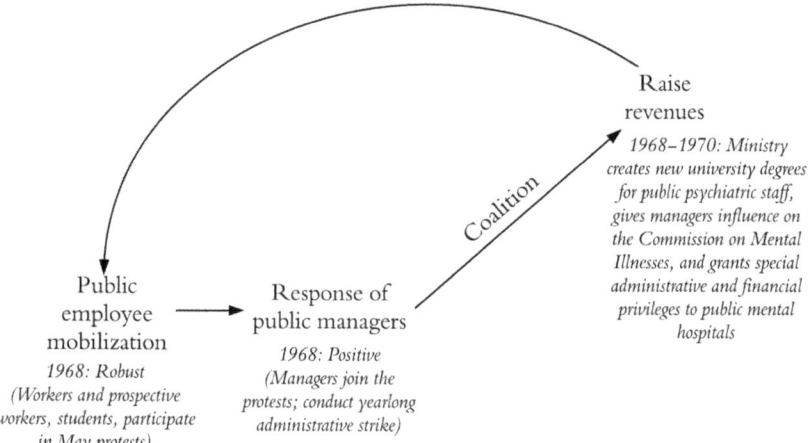

FIGURE 5.2 Second supply-side policy feedback loop, postwar French mental health care

psychiatrists. The subsequent growth of the public mental health workforce, in turn, urged the Syndicat to use these new policy levers to raise revenues for the sectors, positively feeding resources back into the public mental health infrastructure (see Figure 5.2).

1968 Aligns Public Psychiatric Workers and Managers

Prospective Workers Mobilize

The protests of May 1968, though pivotal to the expansion of the public psychiatric workforce in France, remain ingrained in the memories of those outside of mental health as well. Social and economic unrest over the conflict in Algeria, America's growing international influence (especially in Vietnam, a portion of former French Indochina), and labor issues bubbled up as France embarked on its nascent Fifth Republic (Capdevielle and Mouriaux 1988). At the same time, the postwar baby boomers now filled university classrooms, prompting the construction of additional institutions of higher education, the most iconic of which was the University of Nanterre, in the Paris suburbs. In Tilly's (1986, 347) characterization, this "assembly plant for standardized education" offered little in the way of university and research facilities, and even less in the way of future employment prospects.

It is not surprising, then, that it was at Nanterre on May 2, 1968, that the student protests first took hold, before spreading across the Parisian region and throughout the rest of France. The students would be joined by major trade unions, including the CGT and an emerging Socialist affiliate, the French Democratic Confederation of Labor (Confédération française démocratique du travail, hereafter CFDT), and eventually, by an unprecedented number of white-collar workers and employees of high-technology industries too. By May 13, the anniversary of the Algerian rebellion that returned President Charles de Gaulle to power, an estimated 700,000 marchers were protesting in the streets of Paris (Tilly 1986, 343–47).

Pundits often say that little came of this, the largest demonstration in French history. With an angry declaration of "reform, yes, but chaos, no" (*la réforme oui, la chienlit non*), de Gaulle responded by attempting to reorganize government and its leadership. The following year, he invited French voters to reaffirm their commitment to democratic "participation" via a referendum, even though its purposes and promises remained unclear, not to mention mocked by the public. The referendum was the political disaster that ended a two-year struggle by de Gaulle to reassume power. His replacement, Georges Pompidou (who had served as prime minister under de Gaulle), chose to interpret the referendum as a conservative endorsement for decentralization and local government, hardly the radical revolution championed by the protestors (Gourevitch 1980).

Managers Join the Protests

Nevertheless, these events had important implications for the politics of public mental health care in France: A labor–management coalition formed. Initially, the Syndicat distanced itself from the protests, questioning whether its interests would benefit from the generalized chaos (Ayme 1995, 158). Some – including the Syndicat's most celebrated radical, the institutional psychotherapist Dr. François Tosquelles – entirely refrained from taking part.[12] But as the protests/strikes continued, the Syndicat realized the opportunity they afforded. On May 17, the leadership released a press release to "denounce the government repression of student demonstrations." Criticizing first the "archaic structures of education" that had given rise to the protests, the statement then quickly

---

[12] His experience of the Spanish Civil War had made him leery of violent protest, so Tosquelles remained at his home in Melun for the duration of the events of 1968 (Ayme 1995, 156).

returned to its political priorities: "in doing so, [the Syndicat] also denounces the notorious insufficiencies of public health institutions, and of mental health institutions in particular" (Ayme 1995, 159).

The Syndicat's declaration of solidarity with students and workers – broad enough to protect their political independence but militant enough to demonstrate their support – initiated the beginning of a yearlong strike of all administrative duties. While the members of the Syndicat continued their clinical work as physicians, caring for the medical needs of their patients, it was in their capacity as supervisors that they supported the students. Ceasing "all administrative activities" (*tout acte administratif*), they also assembled a national strike committee in charge of organizing local protests that would give the strike a "spectacular and grassroots" (*spectaculaire et populaire*) character. A protest along the Champs-Elysées to the Ministry of Health would amplify their voice further in Paris (Ayme 1995, 182).

Why did the Syndicat agree to form a coalition with workers? Why did it view this moment as a political opportunity? In brief, long-standing challenges to the regulation of hospital psychiatrists' employment could be solved by expanding the public mental health workforce as a whole. To fully understand the Syndicat's involvement in the 1968 protests, one must turn back to a decade earlier, to the law that paved the way for full-time public hospital employment in France. The Law of December 30, 1958, is better known as the "Debré Reform," named for its author, Dr. Robert Debré, a prominent pediatrician from an influential conservative political family. It sought to "rationalize" the country's complex hospital system, boost its research productivity, and promote fairer employment for minorities by offering salaried teaching positions in hospitals located near universities.[13] To top up their salaries, physician-researchers (*universitaires*) at academic medical centers (*Centres hospitaliers universitaires*, hereafter *CHU*) could receive additional payments from patients seeking private consultations, a provision that protected the private practice so closely guarded by the CSMF (CHU Réseau 2008; Rodwin 1982). *Universitaires* could take their public sector salary but still spend significant time attending to privately paying patients in lieu of their other clinical, teaching, and research responsibilities at public hospitals. In other words, the 1958 Debré Reform allowed physicians employed by public (university) hospitals to accept private top-up payments from patients.

---

[13] As a Jewish family, the Debrés were particularly concerned with the residual anti-Semitism of the Second World War (Dutton 2008; Immergut 1992).

Importantly, the 1958 Debré Reform excluded psychiatric hospitals, largely to satisfy the preferences of the Syndicat (Ayme 1995). At the time, a young physician interested in a psychiatric career first would need to obtain a graduate certificate (*Certificat d'études supérieures*, hereafter *CES*) in neuropsychiatry, a discipline that combined neurology and psychiatry, before completing their training in a psychiatric hospital. By contrast, those interested in neurological careers would gain their supplemental training at elite universities and later go on to private practice. At the time of the law's enactment in 1958, the Syndicat expressed concern that merging psychiatric hospitals with *CHUs* could bias students toward neurological careers by limiting their training to the university environment. Training in public psychiatric hospitals would, they feared, become obsolete.[14] Few students would learn about the "specificity" of psychiatry, a notion that helped to both build loyalty to their profession and fill vacant positions at mental hospitals.[15] Participating in the 1958 reform effectively meant surrendering this important staff pipeline, and so this carve-out for psychiatric hospitals was obtained. In short, the 1958 Debré Reform made an exception for psychiatry, so that the discipline would not lose too many students to more lucrative careers in neurology (based in university hospitals).

By the late 1960s, the "double remuneration" problem fostered by the Debré Reform had become a contentious policy issue, one that could be resolved in part by taking advantage of the student protests in 1968. The government decided to "complete" the Debré Reform by definitively splitting private and public hospitals, forbidding those physicians in public, salaried positions from taking any private patients. To encourage young physicians to pursue salaried careers, it expanded the number of positions available at *CHUs*. Thus the incentive formed for the Syndicat: By 1968, the government was willing to spend more money on public university hospital employment to end the use of private payment in that setting.

For mental health workers, both the 1968 student protests and the government's willingness to expand public medical employment offered a unique opportunity to create new degrees and positions in both

---

[14] Note that public psychiatrists also viewed training in university hospitals as "incomplete," precisely because these hospitals did not treat many patients with severe or chronic conditions, contributing to a rival understanding of "mental illness" in that setting. Thanks go to François Chapireau for this point, raised in personal correspondence in August 2023.

[15] Much of Henckes's (2007) analysis centers on the importance of this notion in the development of the French psychiatric profession.

mental hospitals and outpatient sectorized services. The Trade Union of Psychiatric Trainees (Syndicat des psychiatres en formation) advocated for the creation of a separate *CES* in psychiatry, which would definitively prevent them from competing with neurologists in the existing joint program (neuropsychiatry, see Ayme 1995). A similar mobilization supported the efforts of CEMÉA (Centres d'entraînement aux méthodes d'éducation active), the group responsible for the continuing education of social workers, nurses, and other social professions.[16] Although a state-sanctioned nursing degree (*Infirmier d'hôpital d'État*) had existed since 1920, and a special designation for psychiatric nurses (*Infirmiers psychiatriques*) was added in 1955, CEMÉA had sought to establish a more specialized *Infirmier de secteur psychiatrique* (*ISP*) degree following the circular of 1960. This degree would allow for employment growth in the sector as a whole, not only in the hospital. In sum, mental health workers and their managers seized the moment to propose multiple new training pipelines that would encourage workforce growth in public psychiatry.

The 1968 Agreements Expand the Public Mental Health Workforce

It would not be long before the Syndicat's participation in the strike began to yield concessions, the first of which was a new university degree that would significantly expand the mental health workforce. To appease students' requests, legislators enacted a major reform of the university system in November 1968. In December, Education Minister Edgar Faure ordered the creation of a separate *CES* in psychiatry. This, however, was not enough for the protestors. The prestige of this new *CES* relative to the status quo was unclear, and no efforts had been made to accommodate psychiatric nurses' demands for their own *CES*. The strike continued. It was not until May 1969 that the *CES* for sectorized psychiatric nurses (*ISPs*) was granted, nor until September of that year that the government strengthened, via decree, the *CES* for psychiatric physicians.[17]

---

[16] Note that interest in psychiatric work among young '68 protesters is also a reflection of the sociocultural changes of the era. As Henckes (2011b, 175) writes, these professionals were "the avant-garde of a new and rising middle class that promoted human sciences and cultural progressivism throughout society."

[17] See Ayme (1995, 168) and with reference to: Loi 68-978 du 12 novembre 1968 sur l'enseignement supérieur (Loi Faure), Arrêté du 12 mai 1969, Décret du 29 septembre 1969.

These new degrees would boost the pipeline of incoming mental health psychiatrists and nurses. The prestige of the new *CES* remained a significant sticking point. A clause in the decree allowed the *universitaires* to teach in psychiatric hospitals. "It is this last clause that has enraged psychiatric hospital physicians, who had become leery after the many years of domination of their discipline by CHU neuropsychiatrists," reported a 1969 article in *Combat*, a leftist newspaper.[18]

Underlying what Health Minister Robert Boulin called a "doctrinal and emotional" conflict was, of course, an awareness of how these initiatives would impact employment trends.[19] Under the current (1958) law, psychiatrists with research and teaching aspirations had two employment options: the *CHU*, which gave them access to lucrative privately paying patients, or the public psychiatric hospital, where patients were far less affluent and thus these psychiatrists were largely restricted to their salary. The clause in conflict could incentivize psychiatrists to have it both ways (accept private payment in *CHU*s and teach in public psychiatric hospitals), with the effect of depleting psychiatric hospitals of full-time doctors. To express their opposition to the continued "parachuting" of the university physicians out of public psychiatric hospitals, the Syndicat prolonged the strike.[20]

By November 1969, the government had had enough. In a press conference, Health Minister Boulin announced a second concession. To end the strike and resolve the conflict, he would reestablish the Commission on Mental Illnesses, which had been disbanded in 1964. With painstaking attention to maintaining a balance of power, bureaucrats in the Ministry sought to appoint representatives on each side of this public/private dispute. The nomination of the president presented a particular challenge: "It has been customary," the Director General of Public Health, Pierre Boulenger, wrote to Boulin, "that the President alternate between a university physician and a hospital physician." Weighing different options, Boulenger opted to appoint the well-liked hospital psychiatrist Dr. Henri Ey to the presidency and appointed Professor Théophile Kammerer to the vice presidency.[21]

The decision to appoint Henri Ey, "despite his age," to preside over the Commission reveals the desperation of the Ministry. Now in retirement,

---

[18] "Le conflit en psychiatrie: formation d'une commission des maladies mentales," *Combat*, November 7, 1969.
[19] Ibid.
[20] "Le conflit en psychiatrie;" "Création d'une commission de la santé mentale," *Informations médicales*, November 17, 1969.
[21] Although the civil servants were careful in their appointments, the final composition of the Commission favored the *Syndicat* slightly, perhaps in order to repair relations with

Dr. Ey's age should have prevented his involvement in government affairs (he was four years past the age limit for public service). Moreover, his ill health made it more difficult for him to participate. But Ey was a unifying figure; once a president of the Syndicat, Ey had maintained an active neurological research portfolio during his career. The appointment of Professor Kammerer, a university psychiatrist with strong ties to the private sector, as his deputy would help to assuage any concerns regarding Ey's lingering loyalty to the Syndicat, of which he was once president (Garrabé 2005).

Although the appointments of Ey and Kammerer would smooth some tensions over the leadership of the Commission, the question of its membership was just as contentious. Particularly "delicate," as Boulenger put it, was the question of representation by members of the Syndicat.[22] Although Boulenger favored the participation of both para-medical staff (social workers, psychologists, nurses) and nonmedical staff (national public servants, hospital administrators), he worried that "if one admits them all, high-level debates would become but quarrels of influence."[23] He suggested, then, extending ex officio (*à titre de droit*) appointments only to select members, while those with a "special competence in mental hygiene" would be appointed in merely "a personal capacity" (*à titre personnel*). Later that year, the Ministry published an order nominating 44 members to the new Commission, nearly all of whom (41) were appointed in this less formal capacity. Only those organizations who had played a prominent role in the former commission were offered ex officio status: the National Committee for the Prevention of Alcoholism (Comité nationale de défense contre l'alcoolisme), the Autonomous Trade Union of Social Workers in Departmental Services (Syndicat national autonome des assistants sociaux des services départementaux), and the Trade Union of Psychiatric Hospital Physicians (Syndicat des médecins des hôpitaux psychiatriques).[24] The strike ended shortly after this announcement.

---

the strikers. Not only was it presided by Ey, a former president of the trade union, but, in addition, the only physician with an ex officio appointment was Ayme, the current president of the trade union. Moreover, public hospital psychiatrists composed nearly a third of the Commission (14 of 44 members). The ex officio presence of Leclerc as the representative of the social workers' union, furthermore, helped to amplify the voice of other public psychiatric workers as well ("Note pour Monsieur le Ministre" in AN 19910084/28/Réponses à la lettre du 27 mai, 3).

[22] "Note pour Monsieur le Ministre" in AN 19910084/28/Réponses à la lettre du 27 mai, 5.
[23] "Note pour Monsieur le Ministre" in AN 19910084/28/Réponses à la lettre du 27 mai, 5.
[24] Arrêté du 25 novembre 1970: Commission des maladies mentales du conseil permanent d'hygiène sociale, *Journal officiel de la République française*, December 24, 1970.

Even then, the effects of the Syndicat's mobilization carried into the following year. In 1970, legislators finally enacted a third concession: the Second Debré Reform.[25] By formally splitting public and private hospitals, it forbade all public, salaried physicians from accepting privately paying patients. The public designation was extended to psychiatric hospitals, but in order to preserve the "specificity" promised to psychiatric doctors and nurses, a separate hospital category was created: the Specialized Hospital Center (*Centre Hospitalier Spécialisé*, or *CHS*).[26] To accommodate the projected growth in the workforce, the positions of assistant and adjunct *CHS* physicians were added (Leguay 2002, 11; Ayme 1995). This new designation gave mental hospitals significantly more authority over staff training and the distribution of financial resources. This latitude would make it easier for psychiatric hospital administrators to expand sectorized employment, and therefore services, in the coming decade.[27]

Positive Feedback Continues to Expand the Mental Health Workforce and Sectors

The effects of the 1968 protests and the resulting empowerment of mental health workers were evident at both national and local levels. Consider the Syndicat's strategic use of the Commission on Mental Illnesses to rewrite the terms of sectorization in favor of public mental health workers, exemplifying their use of the "brokerage" mechanism. Following the workforce expansions just initiated (and additional agitation by the hospital psychiatrists, who launched a second strike between May and October 1971), the Commission turned to other mental health policy issues by organizing seven different thematic working groups. One group devoted itself entirely to sectorization, another to personnel (AN 19910084/28 and 29). Now that the Syndicat had ensured that few private or university psychiatrists would serve on these subcommissions,

---

[25] Loi 70-1318 du 31 décembre 1970 portant réforme hospitalière, *Journal officiel de la République française*, January 3, 1971, 67–73.

[26] Neurology departments remained attached to *CHUs*. In addition, sectors were "consecrated" as training sites for psychiatric medical students, which helped to build loyalty to the concept (Henckes 2007, 628).

[27] Moreover, the law introduced the concept of a national plan (*carte sanitaire*) that would determine the distribution of hospital beds and equipment throughout the territory. The idea cohered well with the territorial logic of psychiatric sectorization (Jaeger in Reynaud et al. 1994; Leguay 2002; Wilsford 1991).

their public hospital representatives redesigned the Ministry's objectives for the sector. With the help of the Commission, the Ministry released several new documents. The most authoritative was the Order of March 14, 1972, which now required *départements* to participate in sectorization. It was followed by a circular on adult psychiatry that reminded local authorities of the central government funds available (from the May 1955 "social ills" decree) to support the policy.[28]

Most importantly, these documents signaled a shift in tone emblematic of this policy feedback loop. The new circular differed from its predecessor in that it emphasized staff – not buildings – as the core resource of sectorized psychiatry: "Each sector is entrusted to a chief psychiatrist, responsible for a *team* of doctors, social workers, psychologists, nurses, etc." (emphasis in the original).[29] Moreover, the document's annex, "Guidelines Concerning the Sector Team," included an expansive list of professions that should be included in the sector teams: physicians, nurses, social workers, psychologists, even teachers and rehabilitative therapists. This interdisciplinary team would be necessary to "multiply" outpatient services. *Département*-level and hospital administrators were invited to draft a timetable to prepare for the "essential" (*indispensables*) appointments.[30] Over the next two years, a flurry of additional documents and guidelines followed, the last of which concluded that "the years 1972–1973 represented an important stage in the development of French mental health policy."[31]

Throughout the 1970s, medical employment exploded, particularly in psychiatry. As more psychiatrists gained the new *CES* and began new positions as adjunct or assistant *CHS* physicians, they contributed to a ballooning of the number of medical staff at psychiatric hospitals. While the number of psychiatrists in France had hovered around 1,000 in the 1950s, by the 1970s their numbers had reached 13,000 (Cléry-Melin

---

[28] Arrêté du 14 mars 1972, Modalités du règlement départemental de lutte contre les maladies mentales, l'alcoolisme et les toxicomanies (Arrêté du 14 mars 1972), *Journal officiel de la République française*, April 21, 1972, 4206–7; Circulaire 431 du 14 mars 1972 relative au règlement départemental de lutte contre les maladies mentales, l'alcoolisme et les toxicomanies (Ministère de la santé publique et de la sécurité sociale, Direction générale de la santé, Sous-direction de la protection sanitaire, Direction des hôpitaux), *Journal officiel de la République française*, April 21, 1972.

[29] Circulaire 431 du 14 mars 1972, 1.

[30] Ibid., 7.

[31] Circulaire DGS/891/MS 1 du 9 mai 1974 relative à la mise en place de la sectorisation psychiatrique (Ministère de la santé publique et de la sécurité sociale, Direction générale de la santé, Direction de la protection sanitaire), May 9, 1974, 2; see also Circulaire DGS/2030/MS 1 du 12 décembre 1972, Circulaire DGS/1262/MS 1 du 6 juillet 1973, Circulaire DGS/78/MS 1 du 15 janvier 1974 cited in the same.

2002, 796). Similarly, the new *CES* in sectorized nursing generated a steady pipeline of new staff into the growing sectors, as well as of allied mental health providers such as social workers.

As the number of medical degrees and positions proliferated, so too did the trade unions that represented them. The communist union CGT had close ties to public psychiatry through the Syndicat; in its earliest years, many members had been sympathetic to the Communist Party. However, upon its creation in 1964, a union with closer ties to the Socialists, the CFDT, garnered broad appeal among public sector workers, too. Workers who preferred the CGT but rejected the influence of the Communist Party in it, sought representation from the union's offshoot: FO. Unaffiliated trade unions also sprouted during this period. These included the unconventional Trade Union of Psychiatry (Syndicat de la psychiatrie), in which medical professionals advocated "for psychiatry, not psychiatrists" (USP 2021). Motivated to win higher wages, obtain stronger employment protections, and expand their ranks, these trade unions pressured hospital psychiatrists and local administrators to take advantage of sectorization. The availability of the generous May 1955 "social ills" funds – not yet affected by the emerging oil crisis – made it easy to satisfy these pressures. The long-ignored funding mechanism now became central to the maintenance of expanded mental health services (Bauduret 2002).

The national policy changes of this time period were most vividly experienced at the local level. In fact, studies documenting how mental health workers advocated for the expansion of sectorization in individual *départements* has become a rich area of research in recent years.[32] In his study of CGT activists at Le Vinatier hospital and sector in Rhône, Alfandari uncovers a wealth of archival evidence showing how workers advocated for funding increases, staffing diversification and expansion, and secure training and employment schemes in the wake of the post-1968 policy changes. Protecting the sector's public status was also crucial to workers: A joint CGT–CFDT leaflet of 1973 empathically decried "*NON*" to a proposal that would allow private sector organizations to manage some or all sectorized services (reproduced in Alfandari 2017, 91). These efforts are what prompted the local union's then general secretary to claim "'it's thanks to the CGT' that the sector now exists" in an interview years later (quoted in Alfandari 2017, 90).

---

[32] See, for example, Alfandari 2018, Guérin 2011, and the study as part of Gaspard Bouhallier's doctoral thesis, Lumière University, Lyon 2, currently underway at the time of writing.

Local public managers were responsive to such protests, and here, too, acted as brokers between workers and policy-makers. In his study of sectorization in Angers, Vincent Guérin (2011) offers an example that illustrates how public managers took advantage of the generous "social ills" funds to placate their expanding staff. In January 1972, the personnel of the public psychiatric hospital in Sainte-Gemmes-sur-Loire went on strike. The group of protestors, composed mostly of nurses, sought to expand their workforce. In a coauthored report, the *département*'s seven chief psychiatrists (one for each sector) offered their support of the strike, denouncing the fact that it took two protest movements (the first in 1968 and now this one in 1972) to persuade authorities to hire more personnel. To this, they added that the events "could have been avoided if the doctors had been listened to" (Guérin 2011, 498). The timing of the strike, just prior to the collapse of the *Trente Glorieuses*, was fortuitous. The Ministry had just published the March 1972 order and circular, casting renewed attention on the May 1955 funds for social ills. Local authorities quickly complied with strikers' demands, announcing "a happy solution to the conflict through the adoption of exceptional measures and financial means" (Guérin 2011, 498).

The more that policy-makers turned to this financial tool to placate workers, the more the workforce grew. Consider what occurred in Angers over the following decade. Between 1970 and 1977, the number of nurses, caregivers, and social workers (*personnel soignant*) grew from 744 to 992, an increase of more than 30 percent. During this time, the mental health service also added two chief psychiatrists and consequently two medical secretaries. The number of hospital interns almost doubled (from 17 to 31). Spending on nurses alone tripled, taking up an expanding proportion of the *départements*' medical budget (Guérin 2011, 525–26).[33] Moreover, this personnel boom continued even as the number of inpatients was plummeting, from 1,959 to 1,242 (Guérin 2011, 615, table 1).

The second feedback loop therefore demonstrates how intensification of worker demands, engendered by the events of May 1968, prompted public managers to expand the workforce and, by extension, support the expansion of psychiatric sectors. Their proliferation helped to further deinstitutionalization, as they allowed hospitals to more quickly

---

[33] Nurse expenditures increased from around 32 million to 92 million francs during this period. Accounting for the high inflation of the time, these amounts are roughly equivalent to $56 million to $86 million contemporary USD (per INSEE 2023; OECD 2023).

discharge long-stay patients. The coincidence of this period with the *Trente Glorieuses* allowed for the "happy" disbursement of government funds at the local level. Moreover, this economic boom would soon come to an end. The third and final feedback loop shows how the empowered public mental health sector confronted economic crisis.

THE THIRD FEEDBACK LOOP: LONG-TERM, LOCKED-IN FINANCING FOR THE MENTAL HEALTH SECTORS

By the end of the 1970s, public mental health workers and managers discovered that the disbursement of government funds had become decidedly less "happy." In fact, it was downright strained. The oil crisis, combined with a maturing welfare state, put stress on nearly every dimension of the French economy, including the mental health sectors. The election of President Valéry Giscard d'Estaing in 1974 signaled a shift in electoral preferences toward economic conservatism, but it was his prime ministers, Jacques Chirac and especially the economist Raymond Barre, who sought aggressively to reduce government spending in health care through the early 1980s. Hospitals, which comprised more than half of the state's health insurance spending, were a top concern. Significant cost-containment measures followed.[34] When the hospital association claimed that one especially tough motion was illegal, it received a letter from Prime Minister Barre himself buttressing the governments' commitments (Ayme 1995, 340–41).

Mental health care was no exception; if anything, it was more of a target for budgetary cutbacks since its patients tended to lack political influence. Moreover, the 1955 funds for psychiatric sectors remained unstable and insufficient, as the costs of psychiatric hospitals, now inflated by rising numbers of psychiatrists, nurses, and social workers, were increasing. Spending on the sectors became more constrained, and the government announced a target to eliminate 40,000 psychiatric beds (Coffin 2005, 241; Leguay 2002, 14–15). That more young psychiatrists were entering private office practice facilitated this objective and increased public psychiatry's competition from the private sector.

Public mental health workers and managers in France remained united, unlike their counterparts in America, who experienced this period of

---

[34] In 1975, the government began to experiment with a fixed hospital spending growth rate (*taux directeur*) and, in 1978, with global budgeting. The circular of March 29, 1978, set the *taux directeur* at 9.5 percent – a stringent cap when, at the time, the general inflation rate was 17 percent and inflation in health spending was 24 percent (Ayme 1995, 281–82; Leguay 2002, 13–15).

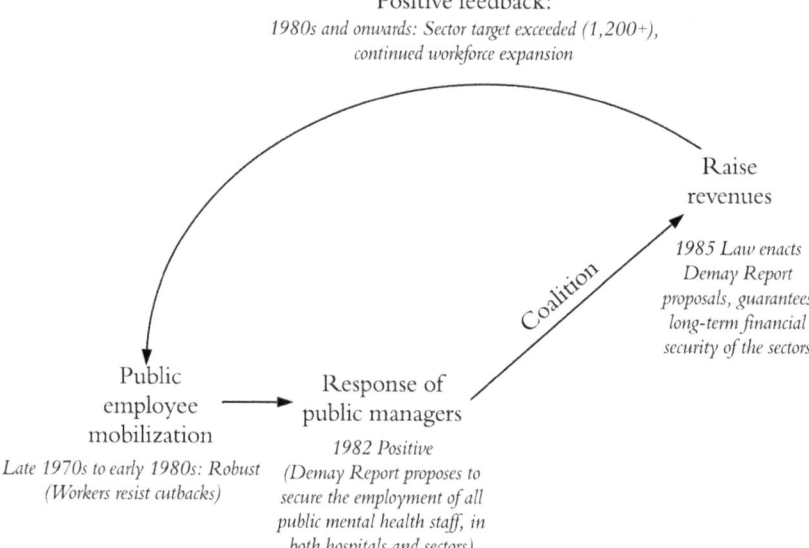

FIGURE 5.3 Third supply-side policy feedback loop, postwar French mental health care

economic retrenchment unaligned. In this third and final feedback loop, this coalition pressured local authorities to maintain sector funding at high levels. Although pressures to cut funds and deinstitutionalize *à l'américaine* by closing hospitals were high, workers and managers jointly stood by a proposal to deinstitutionalize the "French way." In 1985, the government capitulated by securing long-term financing for all public mental health workers and, by extension, for both inpatient and outpatient care. That decision, in turn, has continued to strengthen the power of the public mental health workforce over subsequent decades. The following pages and Figure 5.3 document this positive feedback and Table 5.1 offers a guide to the mental health financing changes it produced.

Public Mental Health Workers and Managers Resist Cutbacks at the Local Level

Despite pressures to reduce financial support for psychiatric hospitals and services, public psychiatry workers in the sectors continued to demand revenue increases from their managers. President Giscard d'Estaing's reforms to health insurance (*assurance maladie*) had slowed, but not halted, hiring in psychiatric services (Ayme 1995, 281–82). Still profiting

TABLE 5.1 *Timeline of psychiatric sector financing in France, key dates*

	The "Sector"			
	Hospital/inpatient services		Non-hospital/outpatient services	
	Payer	Personnel status	Payer	Personnel status
1960–83	Social Security fee-for-service (nondiscretionary)	Social Security (stable)	*Double financement:* state funds for "social ills" and *départements* (discretionary)	DDASS (less stable)
1983–85	Social Security fee-for-service (nondiscretionary)	Social Security (stable)	State funds for "social ills" only (discretionary)	DDASS (less stable)
1985 to present	Social Security global budgeting (nondiscretionary)	Social Security (stable)	Social Security global budgeting (nondiscretionary)	Social Security (stable)

Note: DDASS = Direction départementale des affaires sanitaires et sociales.

from the May 1955 funds for social ills, the sectors remained jointly financed by local health offices (commonly referred to as the Direction départementale des affaires sanitaires et sociales hereafter DDASS) and discretionary central government funds (simply referred to as the State, *l'État*). Moreover, the financial responsibilities of DDASS had lowered to just 17 percent of costs. Observers have remarked that this arrangement, by then referred to as double financing (*double financement*), was "particularly 'heretical,' but of unparalleled efficiency in developing a dynamic public health policy" (Bauduret 2002).

The Managers' Demay Report Proposes a "French" Approach to Psychiatric Deinstitutionalization, with Protections for Public Workers

In 1982, an important window of opportunity opened for public managers to further exert their influence. The defeat of Valéry Giscard d'Estaing by François Mitterrand, a Socialist, ended 23 years of governance by parties of the Right. With Mitterrand's election, the Socialist Party sought to finally implement the "Common Program" (*Programme commun*), a set of Keynesian domestic policies jointly adopted by the Socialist and Communist parties in 1972. When the Socialists released their platform in advance of the election, they had promised to develop sectorization.[35] What is more, shortly after the election, the new Health Minister, Communist Jack Ralite, personally attended the Syndicat's conference in Sotteville-lès-Rouen (October 1981). "Far from suppressing jobs," he declared, "psychiatry must create them."[36]

Proposing that more sectors should be created to support an even smaller catchment area (50,000 people), he concluded with an invitation to the author of a new report:

> For this reason, I entrust to Dr. Jean Demay, known to all for the work he has undertaken in the field of public service psychiatry, a mission of reflection, a mission of invention, to renew psychiatry the French way.[37]

The opportunity to directly influence government policy was welcomed with enthusiasm by the Syndicat and public mental health workers. "We could only rejoice at the Minister's speech," the labor leader Dr. Ayme reflected; "It even went beyond what we had ever dared to claim in terms of the size of the population served by sectors." As for the choice of Dr. Demay, it "deprived us of a member of the union hall in exchange for a reliable and fraternal technical adviser" (Ayme 1995, 375). The next issue of *Vie sociale et traitements* (1981, number 137), the principal journal of sectoral workers, published Ralite's speech in full as its special feature. Mental health workers thus applauded the new government and the auspicious opportunities it offered them (Ayme 1995; Jaeger 1989, 22; Leguay 2002, 15).

Throughout Demay's report, the preferences of public psychiatrists superseded those of private psychiatrists. Typically, the president of the Commission on Mental Illnesses would expect to author a government-mandated report on mental health such as this one. But the Commission presidency had recently rotated to a private psychiatrist, Professor Kammerer. By instead choosing Dr. Demay as the report's author, Minister Ralite ensured that the report would take a public sector approach to mental health provision. For most of the 1970s, Demay had led the Commission's subcommittee on sectorization.[38] Long interested in formalizing the sectorization project into law, he organized a three-day colloquium in 1977 to develop the idea (Leguay 2002, 15). Moreover, the addition of

---

[35] The platform also promised to reform commitment procedures, which remained unchanged since 1838. The Syndicat was less pleased about this; see Club socialiste du livre 1980 in Jaeger (1989, 21).

[36] Jack Ralite, "Déclaration sur la santé mentale" (Sotteville-les-Rouen, October 12, 1981), www.cemea.asso.fr/IMG/pdf/jack_ralite.pdf.

[37] Ibid.

[38] See AN 19910084/28/Groupe de travail secteur.

his wife, Dr. Marie Demay, a pediatric psychiatrist in the public sector, as coauthor of the report contributed further to its public sector orientation (Demay and Demay 1982; Faraggi and Dayot 2016; Leguay 2002, 15).

Contrasting "the French way" of deinstitutionalizing with the British, American, and Italian experiences (see Box 5.1), the Demays (and, by extension, the Syndicat) proposed anchoring their envisioned sectorization project in "public sectoral establishments" (*établissements publics de secteur*). These broadly defined community establishments would assume the responsibilities – and with them, the sustained, stable payment mechanisms – historically associated with mental hospitals. To justify this approach, the Demays looked to their country's long tradition of "great public services, recognized for the importance of their role and the quality of their personnel" (Demay and Demay 1982, 5). This emphasis on personnel reveals much about the agenda driving the report, another tool for brokerage.

Box 5.1 1982 Demay Report Comparative Assessment of the Various "Ways" (*voies*) to Deinstitutionalize

Emphasizing worker protections and service expansions, the 1982 Demay Report proposed a "French way" (*une voie française*) to deinstitutionalize that would differ from that pursued elsewhere:

The English way (*la voie anglaise*): Anti-psychiatry and non-hospital therapeutic communities ... led to very remarkable [community-based] projects. But what became of the movement to close the classic psychiatric hospitals? It seems that the movement, which was very active in the early 1970s, lost its momentum in the context of the economic crisis ... asylums were recreated elsewhere.

The American way (*la voie américaine*): Kennedy's speech (1963) and the social changes of the 1960s and 1970s enabled the mass closure of psychiatric hospitals and creation of community mental health centers. But here also the economic crisis, the abandonment of some former hospital patients, and the [subsequent] violence among some of them obstructed the deinstitutionalization movement. Meanwhile, mental health care appeared to spread into society at large, leading to the insensible psychiatricization of other areas, such as education, law, and prisons.

The Italian way (*la voie italienne*): The radical Law 180 was effective in 4 out of 20 regions, where either the Basaglia movement or sectorization had set up alternatives outside the hospital. Elsewhere, the abandonment of patients, the resistance or sabotage of professional lobbies, and the anguish of families, may perhaps lead to a reform of the law – risking, however, the re-institutionalization of patients in the old psychiatric hospitals.

Source: Demay and Demay (1982, 32)

For many years, sectoral workers had relied on the May 1955 social ills funds to obtain the high revenues necessary for their employment, but the instability of this mechanism prompted a more ambitious agenda: the "unification of personnel statuses" (*unification du statut des personnels*). The segregated financing of psychiatric hospitals (statutorily covered by Social Security) and non-hospital sectoral services (discretionarily covered by the May 1955 social ills funds) had produced two classes of mental health workers: those with positions inside the hospital whose employment could rely on stable Social Security revenues and those positions outside the hospital whose employment depended on the fluctuating social ills funds. (The timeline in Table 5.1 helps to illustrate this division.) While the Syndicat had begun to actively support the unification agenda in the late 1970s, it was through the Demay Report that the managers found an opportunity to communicate those demands to policy-makers most directly (Ayme 1995). By transferring all sectoral services to Social Security, the new establishments would lead to the "disappearance of the current inequalities produced by differences in the authority responsible for payment ... in particular regarding the cases of certain nurses, social workers, psychologists, [and] medical staff" (Demay and Demay 1982, 21). The report was released in July 1982, and in 1983 *Vie Sociale et Traitements* released a full special issue (number 146) celebrating the recommendation. This widespread optimism would, however, soon turn sour in the face of Mitterrand-era austerity measures.

Positive Feedback Develops Legal Protections for Mental Health Sectors, Despite the "Turn to Austerity"

Economic pressures to reduce mental health expenditures reached a tipping point in 1983. The Common Program had failed so spectacularly to meet the standards of the European Monetary System that Mitterrand scrapped the agenda altogether.[39] In a landmark shift known as the "*tournant de la rigueur*" (turn to austerity), the president's branch of the Socialist Party turned away from the Communist and more radical wings of their governing coalition (Levy 1999; Vail 2010). Moreover, the government's tone toward mental health changed substantially. When outlining policy goals in the Ninth Economic Plan (1984–88), Mitterrand

---

[39] The expansionary policies and expensive nationalization measures had deepened the national deficit and reinforced the high inflation rate, while higher taxes had alienated business elites. The franc was devalued three times (OEA 1983).

unveiled a massive reduction target for psychiatric beds that rivaled the aggressiveness of the Reagan and Thatcher administrations abroad: the suppression of 13,000 beds and the conversion of another 28,000 (Commissariat général du Plan 1982; see also Biarez 2004, 517; Coffin 2005, 240; Jaeger 1989, 22). Here was a classic case of crisis-induced deinstitutionalization.[40]

The Syndicat-supported Demay Report would play an important role in protecting mental health workers from Mitterrand's turn to austerity, but at first the Ministry ignored the report. Mitterrand reconfigured his Cabinet, now appointing Edmond Hervé to the Health Ministry. The Commission did not meet for several months. "Rumors emanating from the cabinet suggested that the [new] minister was in favor of this 'hibernation,'" Dr. Ayme (1995, 344) remembers. Moreover, when the Commission eventually convened, the presiding civil servants made no mention of the Demay Report (Jaeger 1989, 22).

Instead, the Ministry privileged the recommendations of another document. Commissioned under the austerity of the previous Barre government and hence published shortly before the Demay Report, the Gallois–Taïb Report (1981, 44–47) had proposed reducing psychiatric services by integrating them into the general hospital system. Although it too denounced the system of *"double financement,"* the Gallois–Taib report argued that the problem could be resolved by relying more on the private, not public, sector. The marginalization of the Demay Report, as Denis Leguay (2002, 17) commented, was "like a sort of burial of the Sotteville speech [by Health Minister Jack Ralite]. Was it too ambitious, [too] costly in terms of human resources?"

Moreover, the laws of January 19, 1983, and January 3, 1984, applied three additional austerity measures to the hospital system by (1) extending the global budget to all *CHU* hospitals, hence (2) formally imposing a fixed hospital spending growth rate (*taux directeur*), and (3) terminating the system of *"double financement"* that allowed both the State and the *départements* to jointly finance services (Safon 2017). The first two reforms, intended for the *CHUs*, did not trouble mental health workers as much as the third. Individual social services (a hospice, a

---

[40] Hospital care was unpopular among some workers, particularly the more radical psychiatrists and psychiatric interns affiliated with the Trade Union of Psychiatry. An open letter to President Mitterrand, published in *Vie sociale et traitements* in 1981, advocated for greater commitments to community care in lieu of hospital care. Syndicat de la psychiatrie, "Lettre ouverte à François Mitterrand, Président de la République," *Vie sociale et traitements* 136 (1981), 42.

rehabilitation center, a clinic) would now receive payments either from DDASS or from the State, but not both. This change gave each payer greater discretion over the services they would choose to fund, prompting the adage "whoever pays, decides" (*qui finance, décide*) and preventing services from using second payers as reinforcements (Reynaud et al. 1994, 255–56). In the area of mental health, the State became responsible for all non-hospital sectoral services, as Table 5.1 shows (Ayme 1995, 247; Bauduret 2002; Leguay 2002, 143). This decision depleted spending on sectoral services by almost a fifth (the 17 percent of costs that had been typically covered by DDASS).[41]

There are different interpretations of what happened next. State policy-makers claimed that the Ministry of Finance never transferred the DDASS funds to the State and refused to finance any spending increases, in order to pressure the Ministry of Health to eventually charge the bill to the Social Security system (Bauduret 2002). Alternatively, mental health professionals rebuked the State's "forgetfulness" as yet another blanket austerity measure (Ayme 1995; Jaeger 1989, 23–25). Regardless of the intent behind policy-makers' forgetfulness, the end result was that the government had reduced financial support for community psychiatry.

It did not take long for mental health workers to respond. With nearly 85 percent of mental health spending going to personnel, the new budgetary reductions forced prefects of the *départements* to terminate contracts, reduce shifts, and forego replacements for outgoing personnel.[42] On June 28, 1985 the Syndicat, the Trade Union of Psychiatry, and the CGT Federation of the Île-de-France (Paris) region, organized a protest in front of the Ministry of Health in Paris (Ayme 1995, 418). At its meeting the next day, the Commission denounced the situation as "perfectly intolerable." The "unilateral decisions" taken by the government had resulted in the "disruption of the entire health care system, challenging jobs and relationships, imposing drastic decisions for budgetary reasons alone, ignoring both needs and technical requirements" (quoted in Ayme 1995, 418).

Upon hearing the statement, the coalition of managers and workers organized an even larger protest on September 20, following it with significant media attention. Hundreds of psychiatrists, psychologists,

---

[41] Monetary estimates of the DDASS deficit vary from about $91 million contemporary USD (Bauduret 2002) to $160 million contemporary USD (Ayme 1995, 399; Jaeger 1989, 25; per INSEE 2023; OECD 2023).

[42] See CFDT statement in Jean-Paul Bossuat, "La psychiatrie à gauche, Vaugrigneuse, les 18, 19, 20 novembre 1981," *Vie sociale et traitements*, 140 (1982), 23–28; see also Ayme (1995); Jaeger (1989, 23–24).

psychometricians, nurses, and social workers protested in front of the ministries responsible for resolving the budgetary "error" (Ayme 1995, 418). In that month's issue of *Vie sociale et traitements*, the CGT, the FO, and the Trade Union of Psychiatry published statements condemning the lack of funds.[43]

That same issue of the journal also explored ways in which the situation could be used to mental health workers' advantage. They had been eyeing the development of global budgeting for several years.[44] Although they were critical of the government's use of the global budget as a tool for austerity, some wondered whether a guaranteed global budget would offer non-hospital sectoral services more stability than the billing per episode that had been in place, especially when "episodes" in community care included relatively inexpensive services such as a group workshop or a short outpatient clinic visit. In a piece entitled "What the Global Budget Could Be," Jacques Ladsous, a special needs educator, reflected on the demerits of the fee-for-service system for mental health care and, in particular, its susceptibility to further retrenchment: "All it takes is to suddenly define 'a day' in a more precise way ... and to demonstrate that a certain number of days were counted unduly. It would be enough, for example, to reduce the notion of 'a day' to the notion of 'accommodation.'"[45]

In short, some mental health workers warmed to global budgeting as payment system that gave them more flexibility than the current fee-for-service system. Although the global budget could be reduced from year to year, the fee-for-service system could undergo more specific and restrictive regulatory changes that would make delivering comprehensive psychiatric services more difficult.

The Ministry seemed to have picked up on some workers' openness toward global budgeting as an opportunity to resolve the "financial stalemate" (*impasse financière*, Bauduret 2002). It returned to the Demay Report, using it now as a template for new legislation that would satisfy both mental health workers and, ironically, the government's austerity program. Here the "adaptive expectations" mechanism discussed in Chapter 1 appears to have been at work. Although this mechanism is perhaps the most difficult to document in the two previous feedback

---

[43] "Des positions syndicales," *Vie sociale et traitements* 154 (1984), 45–46.
[44] The first full issue on the topic appeared in 1979 (number 125).
[45] Jacques Ladsous, "Ce que pourrait être un budget global," *Vie sociale et traitements* 127 (1980), 21.

loops described in this chapter (where only archival and other historical documents are available), I was able to assess its relevance to the third feedback loop by interviewing a former civil servant at the Ministry's Bureau of Psychiatry and lead author of the reforms. The senior official told me that he had drawn on the Demay Report in part because he knew that the prefects feared, above all, the labor protests (*"mouvements sociaux"*) that often came with implementation. The Ministry had long been aware of this concern, having tracked the labor agitation on the ground for at least the last decade.[46] The law that was subsequently proposed, and passed, on December 31, 1985, extended global budgeting to all *CHS* (the public psychiatric hospitals) and included sectorized services as part of that reform.[47] The laws thus "legalized" the sectors by guaranteeing their statutory coverage by Social Security, and in doing so, upgraded the status of sectoral workers outside the hospital (see the last row of Table 5.1).

Through mass mobilization and the strategic use of the Demay Report, therefore, public workers and their organized managers gained a significant concession from a fiscally strained government. The protection and expansion of the public mental health sector was the product of workers' pressure on their managers to expand revenues and protect their employment – pressures that had grown over time and reached their tipping point during this third feedback loop. An independently organized and unified group of public managers, the Syndicat, communicated these demands to government clearly and unequivocally.

Including sectoral services in the *CHS* global budget had important implications for deinstitutionalization. Hospitals had little incentive to increase their inpatient activity. Rather, the prospective global payment encouraged them to re-deploy care to the community setting early and often (Leguay 2002, 21). The result was the accelerated development of diverse, non-hospital sectoral services. By 1989, the country had developed more than 1,000 (Jaeger 1989, 30). Today, France's 1,232 sectors not only meet but in fact exceed the Syndicat's original target (1,200, Chevreul et al. 2015, 147). Their success stands in stark contrast to the intentions and operations of their counterparts in America, presented in Chapter 4.

---

[46] For example, the Commission's archives on sectorization implementation included newspaper clippings from the *F.O. hebdomadaire* (see the October 16, 1976 "Difficultés en psychiatrie et dans les cliniques" in AN 19910084/30).

[47] Loi 85-1468 du 31 décembre 1985 relative à la sectorisation psychiatrique, *Journal officiel de la République française*, January 1, 1986, 7–9.

ALTERNATIVE EXPLANATIONS

I argue in this chapter that the presence of a coalition between public sector workers (e.g., medical interns, nurses, and social workers represented by a wide range of trade unions) and managers (independently represented by the Syndicat) in France produced positive policy feedbacks that gradually increased mental health care services and the overall strength of its workforce. Here I consider three sets of alternative explanations, which are in some ways inversions of the three alternatives explored in the previous chapter on the United States.

Alternative Explanation 1: An Absent Social Movement?

Apart from the 1968 student and labor movement, which benefited the expansion of the public mental health workforce, other social movements are absent from the story of psychiatric deinstitutionalization in France. Public pressure to deinstitutionalize, therefore, seemed limited, in mirror opposition to the American case, where pro-deinstitutionalization sentiment gained strength.

Why is this? The strength of the public mental health workforce, once again, appears to be part of the explanation. If American public mental health workers were not sufficiently powerful to respond to the attacks of those critical of public psychiatry, French workers were just the opposite. A review of the historical evidence suggests that French mental health workers managed to both anticipate and suppress public criticism in ways that ultimately facilitated the expansion of their service.

"Anti-psychiatry" in fact held little sway in France (Henckes 2007, 22). Certainly, France is famous for producing academics who drew on psychiatry and psychoanalysis for their social critiques.[48] But many, if not most, of these thinkers – Michel Foucault, Gilles Deleuze, Félix Guattari, Jacques Lacan, and even the postcolonial theorist Frantz Fanon – positioned themselves more as users, not necessarily critics, of psychoanalytic thought and practice. How society controlled madness, many believed, illuminated numerous questions about the social order. "We are careful not to demand the abolition of these [psychiatric] hospitals," explained a nuanced letter cosigned by Deleuze, Lacan, and others,

---

[48] As Goldstein (1987) writes in her preface, French bookstores can house entire sections devoted to "anti-psychiatry."

published in *Le Monde*.[49] Only a few radical offshoots of those critics (e.g., the Foucauldian-inspired Asylum Information Group, or Groupe information asiles) seriously engaged the question of whether the entire psychiatric system should be overturned.[50] In broader public discourse, that question never quite materialized.

Public psychiatrists, for their part, preempted it with a coherent response. In the mid 20th century, many psychiatrists were themselves deeply critical of the social control functions of the psychiatric institution. For example, in a series of writing produced in the 1970s, Henri Ey and his colleagues expressed their shock at being considered "jailers" in the country where Philippe Pinel famously freed the mentally ill from their chains (Coffin 2005, 240). For reasons such as this one, public psychiatrists developed their "institutional psychotherapy" method (described in Chapter 3) to promote more social forms of treatment – but from within the walls of the public mental hospital.[51] Thinkers such as Guattari and Fanon trained precisely at the hospital where "institutional psychotherapy" first emerged (St. Alban), rendering them even more likely to support this method. It helped to lay the intellectual foundation for the sectorization policy, which some even framed as a form of antipsychiatry itself (Martin 2004).

To be sure, psychiatrists were not immune to criticism after institutional psychotherapy developed, including from some of their own coalition partners. At a conference of the Syndicat in 1974, a collective of nurses and other mental health professionals presented a 310-page report

---

[49] Marie-Claire Boons, Guy Clastres, Denise Demoy, Françoise Dolto, Laurence Friedmann, Francis Hofstein, Irène Kotsonis, Jacques Lacan, Lucien Melèse, Jeanine Mouchonnat, Michèle Montrelay, Philippe Rufenacht, François Raux-Filio, Christian Simatos, Bernard This, Radmilla Zygouris, Gilles Deleuze, "Correspondance: l'Antipsychiatrie," *Le Monde*, March 12, 1971.

[50] Furthermore, it was not until decades later that this group would make a dent in French mental health policy. Advocacy by the Asylum Information Group before the French Constitutional Court contributed to the passage of a 2011 law guaranteeing systematic judicial reviews of involuntary care after a predetermined period of hospitalization (15, then 12, days; see Barnard 2019b). Compare this late and limited liberalization of commitment practices in France to its much earlier and more substantial counterpart in the United States, where activists faced less opposition (described in Chapter 4).

[51] From a cross-national standpoint, mental health care systems appear to reinforce certain psychotherapeutic philosophies, and vice versa. Where public funding for mental health care is generous, as in France and Norway, psychiatrists have tended to develop and emphasize the social dimension of care. Where public funding for mental health care is limited, as in the United States and Sweden, psychiatrists have tended to emphasize a biomedical tradition. By applying a comparative, historical, and political-economic lens to mental health care, this book can help to explain how such complementarities came about.

exposing psychiatrists' demagoguery. (That these groups formed alliances in politics does not mean that they always got along in the workplace.) Soon thereafter, the public accused the Syndicat, with its historical ties to the French Communist Party, of sympathizing with Soviet psychiatry and its full range of horrors. At its 1978 conference in Deauville, the Syndicat developed a broad public relations strategy to respond to these critiques. The 300 participants assembled to recast the union as both a scientific and a labor organization and to formulate a coherent intellectual response to their critics that justified the protection of public psychiatric services (Ayme 1995, 326–27). The papers presented emphasized the therapeutic justification for public psychiatry, extending and rejuvenating the concept of sectorization to refute its harshest critics. Through a series of promotional events and press – both in France and overseas – they worked to distance themselves from the Soviet Union and authoritarian approaches to psychiatry as a whole.[52]

With the exception of the collective just described, however, mental health workers generally contributed to efforts to refute anti-psychiatric critiques. Union activists combined an intellectual reframing of anti-psychiatry with cunning mobilization strategies. Drawing on both archival sources and oral histories, Alfandari (2017, 2018) examines how CGT militants defined themselves as both political leftists who opposed the authoritarian "asylum" and loyal employees of the publicly funded sectors. Meanwhile, Bouhallier (2021) has discovered archival evidence that unions actively mobilized patients and their families to contest hospital closures in the postwar period. In other words, the unions representing mental health workers played a direct role in amplifying client demand for services and support for the psychiatric establishment. Together, public psychiatric workers and managers reinforced a mental health policy paradigm that made little room for anti-psychiatric critiques.[53]

Alternative Explanation 2: The Central Authority of *l'État*

Over the second half of the 20th century, France's powerful and centralized *État* (State) appeared to become even more so. Gaullist public policy

---

[52] See, for example, Ayme's (1995, 240, 277) discussion of the Mexico conference and writings of journalist Claire Brisset (daughter of Syndicat member Dr. Charles Brisset): "L'Association mondiale de psychiatrie renouvelle sa condemnation des pratiques abusives," *Le Monde*, July 9–10, 1977; "Psychiatrie et politique," *Le Monde*, August 27, 1977.

[53] This political sociology resembles closely what Bergeron (1999) has theorized and described in the case of French substance abuse policy.

adopted a top-down, *dirigiste* approach to managing the economy, which a commanding bureaucracy implemented. This approach may have advantaged the French public mental health workforce, which unlike its American counterparts faced fewer institutional veto points that checked its influence. Personal accounts of how the 1960 administrative circular came to be illustrate this pattern. The bureaucrats' influence was notable. Their Parisian office, Dr. Ayme's memoir recalls, "was the control tower for all of psychiatry in France and its overseas territories" (Ayme 1995, 52). Once the Syndicat gained the ears of the bureaucrats, though, these policy-makers were "conquered by the idea of the sector" (Daumezon in Murard and Fourquet 1975, 185).

Recall, though, that State bureaucrats were unsuccessful at implementing sectorization policy during the first feedback loop. Even if the Ministry did come to support the policy in the 1960s, the fact remains that few sectors developed at the height of *dirigisme*. This "long sleep" lasted until 1968. At that point, managers and workers allied to expand public employment opportunities in public psychiatry as a whole. Only afterwards did sectors proliferate.

State enthusiasm for sectorization then cooled during the second feedback loop, just as services expanded. While health care cost containment was becoming a priority in Paris, *départements* were turning to the "social ills" funds to increase mental health care expenditures. This conflict between national and subnational levels of government belies stereotypes of France's unitary government structure. The reality is more complicated. Mental health workers and managers lobbied across a range of local institutions and their representatives, including elected officials on departmental councils (*conseils généraux*, or *conseils départementaux* as of 2015), mayors heading municipalities, as well as local labor dispute settlement and planning bodies (e.g., *commissions paritaires départementales, comités techniques*).

The incentives of policy-makers in these local institutions differed from those of their counterparts in Paris. Public psychiatric services were "a bit like the mine of the region, the big company around which the village economy revolved."[54] Local leaders were concerned about maintaining local employment and could exploit central funds to do so. Moreover, left partisans have historically been very responsive to local public sector trade unions, granting them much more power in some

---

[54] Thanks go to Gaspard Bouhaillier for this language, cited from personal correspondence in December 2023.

regions compared to others (Vincent 2016), and even compared to the national level. Indeed, unions in France have less direct influence on national policy than their counterparts in textbook corporatist countries such as Germany. But again, local incentives differ, in ways that in the 1970s benefited local mental health workers.[55]

The financial strain and austerity policies of the 1980s made the State even more committed to cost containment during the third feedback loop (Bauduret 2002). It attempted, but did not fully succeed, to make drastic cuts to psychiatric services. Rather, the State agreed to a compromise proposed by the coalition itself. The following section will consider to what extent this compromise was part of the broader economic plans of that decade; however, it is unlikely that sectors would have gained national attention had they not already become staples of local economies in the previous decade. In some ways, sectors had developed against the prerogatives of the otherwise powerful *État*.

Alternative Explanation 3: The Role of Public Employment in the French Political Economy

French policy-makers have often expanded public employment for strategic political and economic reasons. After 1968, the new public sector positions would help to satisfy young protestors' demands for employment. In the 1980s, the Mitterrand government restricted public employee wages to achieve the fiscal austerity and internal devaluation required by the European Monetary System, while also adhering to the Socialist government's political commitment to Keynesian-style full employment. To compensate for the high unemployment of this period (exacerbated by the restructuring and industrial sector layoffs that followed the oil shocks), French policy-makers expanded public – albeit low-paid – employment (see Di Carlo 2023, also confirmed in personal communication). To what extent can these political strategies explain the expansion of public mental health employment? To what extent did the advocacy of the welfare workforce, especially in mental health care, shape those outcomes?

---

[55] This local-level activity in fact accords with another prominent public policy approach in France at that time. For example, and as mentioned earlier in this chapter, President Georges Pompidou, developed a robust localist agenda that formed the basis of later efforts to "de-concentrate" French social services (Cole 2008). Although these services were managed and organized in Paris, significant local activity would determine their distribution on the ground.

Not all segments of the public sector workforce benefited equally from these targeted expansions.[56] Perhaps the most illustrative contrast comes from disability policy, a close cousin of mental health care but, in this case, also its competitor. Over the latter half of the 20th century, services for people with physical disabilities developed a private, not-for-profit, and targeted character, never gaining the full Social Security coverage that the public and universal mental health sectors did (Barnard 2019a, 766). Had French policy-makers sought to expand public employment irrespective of workers' demands, one would expect similar policy outcomes in the disability sector as in mental health care. But that did not occur.

This divergence is partly attributable to the strength of public mental health professionals, who in effect feared losing their clients to another social sector. Note that the cards were stacked against them. In 1975, an association representing the families of people with mental illness managed to get a law passed that encouraged the transfer of residents of mental hospitals into the not-for-profit "*médico-social*" sector.[57] But two articles of this law were particularly troubling to public psychiatric workers. Article 46 established separate services for the care of "dependent adults with chronic medical needs," and Article 47 promised a decree detailing the conditions under which the State would cover "the expenses incurred in establishments receiving mentally ill persons whose condition no longer requires care in a psychiatric hospital but does require temporary medical supervision."[58]

The public mental health workforce responded by actively opposing those provisions, and they succeeded. Scholarly accounts point

---

[56] By some accounts, the French form of neoliberalism may even have hit hardest in the public sector labor force, where the size of the state declined over the long term (Prasad 2006, 235).

[57] UNAFAM (then shorthand for Union de familles de malades mentaux et de leurs associations, or the Union of Families of the Mentally Ill and their Associates) was the major representative of people with severe and chronic conditions in France at this time. It was founded in 1963, sixteen years earlier than its counterpart NAMI (then the National Alliance for the Mentally Ill) was founded in the United States. This earlier start allowed UNAFAM to participate in the overall trajectory of deinstitutionalization more than NAMI, though the record of its success is mixed. Note also that UNAFAM and NAMI originated as parents' associations and hence held policy positions that may have differed from those of the mentally ill themselves (see Chapter 1). In recent years, NAMI has made efforts to shift its focus from families to people with mental illness.

[58] Loi 75-534 du 30 juin 1975 d'orientation en faveur des handicapés and Loi 75-535 du 30 juin 1975 relative aux institutions sociales et médico-sociales, *Journal officiel de la République française*, July 1, 1975, 6596–6607.

unequivocally to how powerful public psychiatrists, in particular, shaped this outcome (Barnard 2019a, 2019b; Henckes 2007, 2011a, 2011b). The profession would play an important role in defining the disabled, as doctors have in other countries (Stone 1984). But notice that French psychiatrists had specific economic interests at stake. Debates from the Syndicat's 1978 Deauville conference – one already sensitive to employee demands – reveal the managers' concerns about the potential for service competition (as opposed to the eligibility criteria of insurance benefits). One important paper proposed adding "intermediary structures," a public sector alternative to those proposed in the 1975 disability law, to the sectors.[59] In particular, "therapeutic apartments" would shift patients from the hospital setting to a less medicalized, more community-oriented one.[60] These facilities were anchored firmly in the public sectorization system and offered more job opportunities for their sectorized employees than for themselves. (Such services are far less medicalized, and thus less dependent on physicians, than hospitals and outpatient clinics.) By the end of the 1978 conference, the Syndicat had passed several new resolutions. They denounced the disability law's "serious risks of developing a network of institutions parallel to the public service" and renewed "its demands for 'a financial tool' that would be adapted to the situation" (Ayme 1995, 328). To date, those resolutions have been largely reflected in public policy: The comprehensive set of mental health sectors gained stable Social Security coverage in 1985, while disability services remain privately provided and less generously funded.

This 1985 law, it should be added, achieved goals different from those of French macroeconomics at that time. Although the Mitterrand government prioritized young people entering the labor market for the first time, the 1985 law that legalized mental health sectors primarily affected those already employed. In fact, it did more to strengthen existing public sector jobs (by converting *département*-run outpatient care into more stably financed services) than expand them. This outcome, too, was the direct result of the advocacy of the welfare workforce. The Mitterrand government may have sought to expand public employment overall, but

---

[59] See Dameron and Reverzy paper in Ayme (1995, 328).

[60] The group even debated whether the hospital was necessary to the sector at all. While some argued that sectorization, as originally conceptualized by Bonnafé, did require hospital care; others argued against that idea. See the Berthelier–Constant–Karavokyros debates in Ayme (1995, 328).

in mental health care it did so according to the specific terms set forth by the public labor–management coalition in that sector.

Certainly, not all has been positive in French mental health care since 1985. Coordination with the disability sector, ironically, has become a challenge. Austerity measures have made it difficult for outpatient services to meet demand, especially for psychotherapy. They have also incentivized staff flight to the private sector, not unlike the "YAVIS" phenomenon described in the previous chapter did in the United States (Bauduret 2022).[61] Although the overall financial structure and universality of the French mental health system has not been seriously challenged, it is notable that these strains began to appear as psychiatric management fragmented. At least four other unions of hospital and sector psychiatrists have emerged (Karavokyros 2010). Moreover, public managers trained in medicine, previously represented exclusively by the Syndicat, are less the norm now than before. The 2010 creation of regional health agencies (*agences régionale de santé*), as Tartour (2021) has highlighted, deepened the fragmentation of the mental health care administration as well. These divisions may make coalition formation and continued advocacy for service expansion more difficult for mental health workers, even if their primary employment protections have long been secured.

In comparative perspective, though, the "French way" of deinstitutionalizing psychiatric services produced higher levels of public mental health care than in many other countries. One cannot explain this contemporary outcome without acknowledging the historical role of the welfare workforce. A coalition of workers and independently organized, unified managers advocated to develop, expand, and ultimately sustain mental health sectors, the diversified set of services that would complement institutional care. That public mental health care withstood austerity, though, is not unique to France. The next chapter shows how a similar pattern shaped the expansion of services in Norway and its absence facilitated their decline in Sweden, as they did in the United States. This shadow case comparison of two otherwise generous social democratic welfare states can assess whether and how the argument presented in this book generalizes to other countries.

---

[61] In fact, financing psychotherapy is a major mental health care policy challenge across the affluent democracies. The YAVIS phenomenon helps to explain why. But in addition, policy-makers have been reluctant to fund a technique with higher labor costs and less scientific backing than psychopharmaceuticals and other biomedical alternatives. Conflicts over who can provide talk therapy have also impeded public coverage (as has been the case in France).

TABLE 5.2 *Within-case process-tracing tests, France*

Empirical questions (and type of process-tracing test, Van Evera 1997; Bennett 2010)	Evidence	Interpretation
Core theoretical argument 1: Public sector workers and managers express the same preferences for public service maintenance and expansion.		
1.A. Do workers mobilize in favor of public service maintenance and expansion? (Hoop test)	Mobilization at the local level, for example, in the Seine *département* during the first feedback loop (hospitals only); 1968 protests at the national level and subsequent mobilization at the local level, for example, Rhône, Angers, during the second feedback loop (sector-wide); mobilization in the early 1980s during the third feedback loop (sector-wide). Role of Syndicat in Debré Reforms (1958, 1970) and Demay Report (1982).	Yes, public psychiatric workers (in both hospitals and sector-wide) regularly mobilized in favor of public service maintenance and expansion throughout deinstitutionalization.
1.B. Does an independent and united organization of public sector managers allow them to express a preference for public service maintenance and expansion? (Hoop test)		Yes, an independent and united organization of public psychiatric managers allowed them to express (and defend) their opinions separately from the private sector.
1.C. Do workers and managers form a coalition? (Hoop test)	Joint statements and mobilization at national level (1968, 1985) and in *départements* (e.g., Seine in the first feedback loop, Angers in the second feedback loop).	Yes, public sector workers and managers formed coalitions at the national and local levels during deinstitutionalization.

(continued)

153

TABLE 5.2 (continued)

Empirical questions (and type of process-tracing test, Van Evera 1997; Bennett 2010)	Evidence	Interpretation
Core theoretical argument 2: The coalition of public sector workers and managers procures concessions from policy-makers by way of the following causal mechanisms:		
2.A. Brokerage: Do public managers use the privileged tools at their disposal to secure and expand the delivery of public services? (Smoking-gun test)	Role of public managers on the Commission on Mental Illnesses/Health, in departmental councils (e.g., Angers example), and in the Demay Report.	Yes, public managers brokered the demands of workers (and advocated for their own) throughout deinstitutionalization.
2.B. Adaptive expectations: Do policy-makers make concessions because they fear retribution from the coalition? (Smoking-gun test)	Rationale stated by senior French civil servant in interview for the 1985 legislation; see also the statements and actions of Boulin and Boulenger in 1969 and local authorities in Angers in 1972.	Policy-makers expressly feared retribution from workers during the third feedback loop. Statements and actions of policy-makers during the second feedback loop, as well as the evidence in 1.C and 2.A, implies that a coalition with managers augmented that threat.
Core theoretical argument 3: Positive feedback reinforces the coalition, relaunching the feedback cycle.		
3.A. Does the public sector workforce expand as funds for public services increase? (Hoop test)	Expansion after the 1968–72 national policy changes, and continued growth as workers begin to leverage "social ills" funds at the local level.	Yes, the public sector psychiatric workforce expanded over successive feedback loops.

3.B. Do workforce mobilizations become more robust as funds expand? (Hoop test)	Limited mobilization in the first feedback loop, followed by more robust mobilization at the local level in the second feedback loop, culminating in the national protests in the third feedback loop.	Yes, the mobilization of public sector psychiatric workers became more robust over successive feedback loops.
Alternative explanations:		
Alt.A. Did the absence of a pro-deinstitutionalization movement in France independently lead to the expansion of public mental health care?	Both public psychiatric managers and workers actively refuted anti-psychiatric critiques in favor of protecting public revenues for their services. (Passes a doubly-decisive test standard)	No, the absence of a pro-deinstitutionalization movement was at least in part the result of worker–manager advocacy in mental health care.
Alt.B. Did the powerful and centralized French State independently lead to the expansion of public mental health care?	The timeline of sectoral development does not align with the timeline of the State's prerogatives. (Passes a hoop test standard)	No, the nature of the French State did not over-determine the success of the labor–management coalition in this policy area.
Alt.C. Did French policy goals independently lead to the expansion of public mental health care employment?	A comparison between the mental health and disability sectors reveals that policy-makers protected and expanded public services in the former more than in the latter, in part because of the advocacy of mental health professionals. (Passes a smoking-gun test standard)	No, employment in public mental health care did not increase simply because increasing public employment overall was a national policy goal.

6

Deinstitutionalization Elsewhere

A Scandinavian Check

The preceding chapters have shown how welfare workers shape the welfare state by tracing their influence on the development of mental health care in the United States and France. Despite initially similar conditions in the two countries, postwar public mental health employees in America were not able to form coalitions with their managers, while those in France were successful at doing so. This difference produced contrasting cycles of negative and positive supply-side policy feedback in mental health care in the second half of the 20th century – precisely when policy-makers sought to "deinstitutionalize" the mentally ill out of hospitals, partly to reduce costs (see Figure 6.1). While France maintained and expanded the supply of public mental health care services even as psychiatric deinstitutionalization progressed, the absence of political pressure from their American counterparts facilitated the opposite result in the United States. A half-century after the push for deinstitutionalization, the supply of mental health care in France is nearly three times that of the United States (see Figure 6.2).

Although much can be learned by contrasting these paradigmatic and influential cases, some questions nevertheless remain. To what extent did the generosity of the French welfare state, with its emphasis on state welfare provision, tilt the trajectory of mental health care in that country toward robust public provision? To what extent did the fragmentation of American society – racial and governmental – curtail the possibilities for social solidarity in this policy area? To what extent are these outcomes attributable more to the varying strengths of the labor movements in each country than to the coalitions of public workers and managers in mental health? And, in the case of mental health policies developed in the 1970s and 1980s, to what extent did public managers' secondary identities as

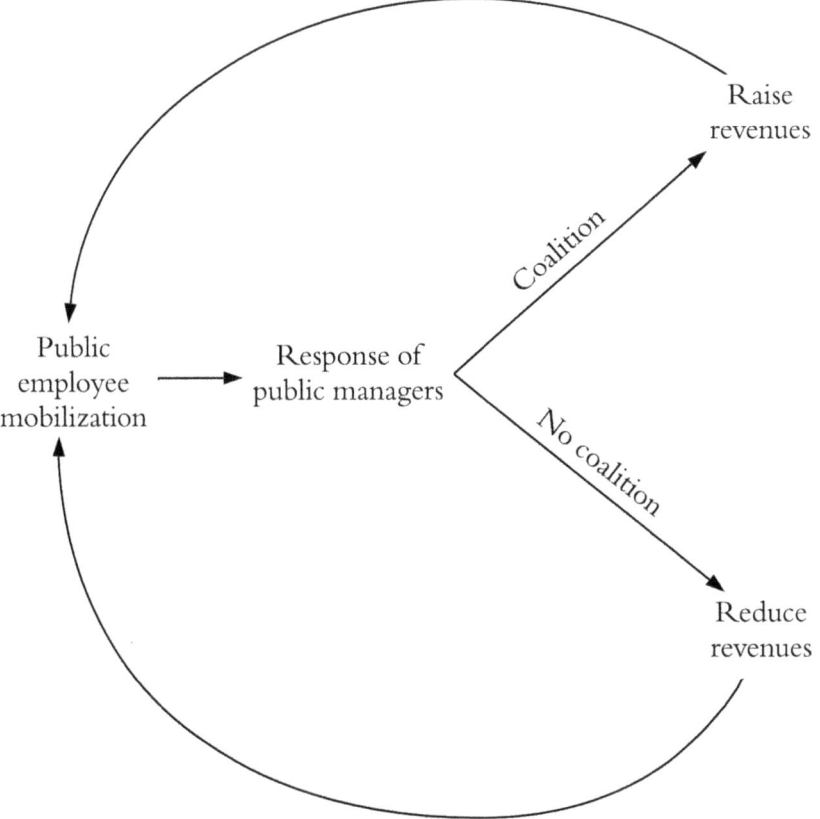

Positive feedback:
more public services, employment security and
protections, workforce growth, support for labor rights

Raise
revenues

Coalition

Public
employee
mobilization

Response of
public managers

No coalition

Reduce
revenues

Negative feedback:
fewer public services, reduced wages and
protections, layoffs, less support for labor rights

FIGURE 6.1 Supply-side policy feedback model: Effects of public sector worker alliances on the supply of public social services for disenfranchised populations (basic diagram of theoretical argument)

psychiatrists shape their preferences and political influence? The previous chapters have addressed these alternative explanations through both structured comparison and within-case process analysis; however, the evidence has been limited to the French and American cases, that is, to the countries that produced those questions in the first place.

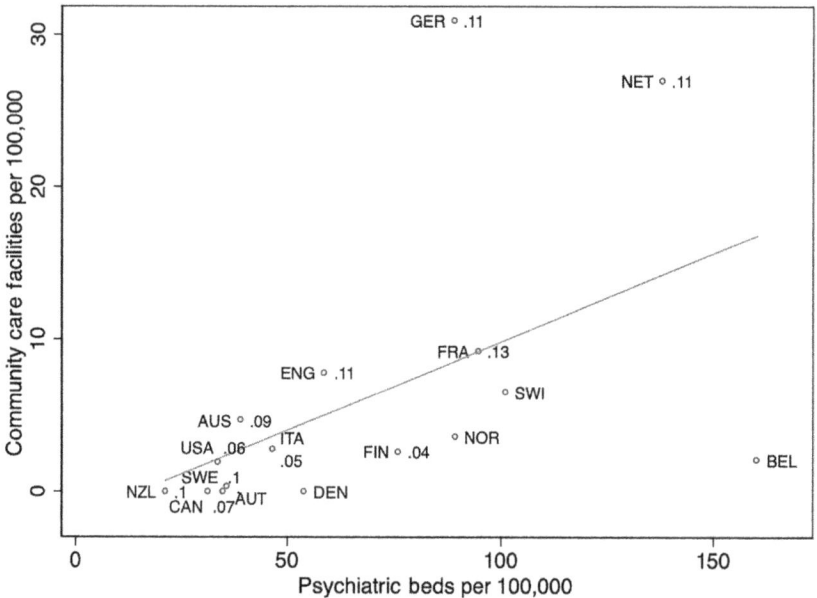

FIGURE 6.2 Scatterplot of psychiatric beds and community care facilities per 100,000 in 16 high-income democracies, with percentage of health budget allocated to mental health (as available) and line of best fit
Source: WHO (2011)

Another way to assess the causal importance of these lingering questions is by testing the argument outside of the primary comparative cases. This chapter offers that analytic check. I examine whether and how coalitions within the welfare workforce shaped policy feedback in mental health care in Sweden and Norway. These two Scandinavian societies share much in common that control for the above explanations: statist welfare provision, ethnic homogeneity, a long history of social solidarity, and a powerful trade union movement (see Mill 1874; also Slater and Ziblatt 2013; Tarrow 2010). Yet when it comes to mental health care, these two cases are polar opposites. Norway's supply of mental health care is significantly higher than that of Sweden (see Figure 6.2), whose dramatic reduction of psychiatric care in the 1990s in fact paralleled that of the United States earlier in the century. Evaluating the external validity of the argument in these two "shadow cases," then, can determine its robustness (see Soifer 2020). Moreover, the selection of these two cases can assess whether the argument "travels" across all three "types" of welfare states: liberal (United States), conservative (France), and social democratic (Norway and Sweden) (see Esping-Andersen 1990). The following pages first introduce Sweden and Norway's mental health systems and their similar starting points; then present evidence documenting the supply-side policy feedback theory at work in each case; and close by assessing the major alternative explanations, including the counterargument that Norway's access to rich oil revenues overdetermined the policy outcomes in that country. But as the evidence nonetheless shows, the presence of a coalition between managers and workers in Norway and its absence in Sweden indeed played a role in their diverging approaches to psychiatric deinstitutionalization.

DIFFERENT OUTCOMES, SIMILAR SOCIETIES

The differences observed between Sweden and Norway in Figure 6.2 emerged only at the very end of the 20th century (compared to France and the United States, where the divergence began decades earlier). In the 1990s, Sweden and Norway each underwent significant reforms in their mental health care sector, with opposite results. Their initial aims matched the deinstitutionalization reforms in other countries, including those of France and the United States in prior decades (see Chapters 4 and 5). As elsewhere, deinstitutionalization in Scandinavia first began in the mid 20th century, when the postwar expansion of the welfare state rendered life outside the "asylum" possible for its residents (see Chapter 2). But it was not until the 1990s that the governments of Sweden and Norway took formal steps to make this process national policy.

Under the 1995 Psychiatry Reform, the Swedish Parliament (*Riksdag*) amended preexisting legislation (the Social Services Act) to formally devolve responsibility for the nonmedical care of the mentally ill (i.e., social services, such as housing and employment services) from the county to the municipal level. The logic of this decision will be familiar to readers by now, as doing so would allow the country to depopulate its county-level mental hospitals (until then, the default custodians of the long-term mentally ill). To facilitate this transition, the central government provided the municipalities with a short-term implementation grant: 1.2 billion Swedish krona over a two-year period (about $200 million contemporary USD; per OECD 2023; SCB 2023). As a result, the patient population residing in county hospitals plummeted by a third, but relatively few municipalities developed sufficient compensatory social services (Malm et al. 2002; Silfverheim and Kamis-Gould 2000). These outcomes have garnered the 1995 reforms a public reputation as a "policy failure," or in the poignant words of the leading Social Democratic politician Lars Engqvist, a "disgrace for Sweden."[1]

On the heels of that Swedish reform, in 1996–98, the Norwegian Parliament (*Storting*) opted for a different approach to a similar policy problem. To deinstitutionalize the mentally ill living in its county-level long-term care institutions, Norway repurposed some of those facilities. Psychiatric nursing homes became outpatient "district psychiatry centers" (*distriktspsykiatrisk senter*). Moreover, Parliament provided ample funds to both county and municipal governments to develop other services for people with mental illness via a decade-long "Escalation Plan." The funds, which in total amounted to 24 billion Norwegian krone (or about $5 billion contemporary USD; per Norges Bank 2023b; OECD 2023) disbursed over eight years, allowed local governments to develop longer-term plans, including those that required hiring new personnel. The funds would go further in Norway, too, as its population was about half that of Sweden's. Indeed, the outpatient mental health care workforce doubled during this time (Romøren 2018). The effects of this initiative on the supply of mental health care in Norway therefore were quite different than in Sweden's case. Between 1998 and 2007, inpatient care declined by 1,800 beds (mostly in psychiatric nursing homes), but it was fully replaced – even exceeded – by 1,865 new places in the outpatient district psychiatry centers and a range of new ancillary services. A direct benefit to mental health workers, further, was the rise in staffing levels: about a 20 percent increase overall and doubling in the outpatient setting alone (Romøren 2018). Table 6.1 summarizes the main differences between Norwegian and Swedish mental health policy outcomes.

That Sweden and Norway diverged so much on the deinstitutionalization of mental health care is surprising because, prior to these reforms, their systems were very similar. As is evident from Table 6.2, in 1990 the population-adjusted supply of psychiatric care was almost identical in both countries. The distribution of these services varied only slightly. Sweden provided more inpatient care in hospitals (mental and general) than Norway, where psychiatric nursing homes often offered that care instead. Note that the size of the mental health workforce was similar, too (see Table 6.3). Although Norwegian psychiatric nurses outnumbered their Swedish counterparts, the density of other mental health care professionals was about the same in the two countries.

---

[1] Lars Engqvist, interview, *Aktuellt*, Sveriges Television, January 3, 2000.

TABLE 6.1 *Divergent results of mental health policy reforms in Sweden and Norway in the 1990s*

	Sweden	Norway
Expenditures committed	1.2 billion SEK (about $200 million contemporary USD) over two years, for population of 8.8 million	24 billion NOK (about $5 billion contemporary USD) over eight years, for population of 4.4 million
Inpatient mental health care	Most county-level hospitals eventually close	No hospital closures (only psychiatric nursing homes downsized)
Outpatient mental health care and social supports	Limited (e.g., about 60 sheltered housing projects created in total)	Extensive (e.g., creation of District Psychiatry Centers, with over 1,800 new places and ancillary services)
Staffing	Overall de-professionalization of the workforce; no training programs; precise numerical data not available, though sources imply limited to no growth	Significant growth (doubled in the outpatient setting; by 20 percent sector-wide); large-scale training and upskilling programs

TABLE 6.2 *Supply of mental health care in Sweden and Norway prior to the reforms (vårdplatser, "care places" – or beds and patient spots – per 100,000 population in 1989–90)*

	Sweden	Norway
Mental hospitals	64	57
Psychiatric wards in public hospitals	50	30
Psychiatric nursing homes	70	100
Other	6	6
Total	190	193

Source: SOU 1992:4, 57

Beyond supplying similar levels of care, the two countries also administered this care in parallel ways. Both Sweden and Norway tasked their counties with administering the medical arm of mental health services, while their municipalities addressed the social arm (e.g., housing, employment support, daytime assistance). Centralized public financing paid for the medical arm of services and municipal taxes financed the

TABLE 6.3 *Mental health care workforce in Sweden and Norway prior to the reforms (per 100,000 population in 1989–90)*

	Sweden	Norway
Psychiatrists	10	9.6
Psychologists	9	9.7
Nurses	51	91.2
Social workers	9	8.1
Other	245	248.8
Total	324	367.4

Source: SOU 1992:4, 58

social arm.[2] As for private mental health care, a combination of patient fees and social insurance funds financed the few private services that existed in each of these countries.

When each country set out to reform mental health provision in the early 1990s, their aims were similar too. As in other countries, the advent of antipsychotic medications and critiques of the psychiatric hospital (and professional discipline) had spurred public support for deinstitutionalization (Diseth 2017; Ohlsson 2008). Economic constraints also motivated deinstitutionalization in Scandinavia – especially in Sweden, which faced a more severe financial crisis than Norway at the time. Norway would both recover from its crisis more quickly and, around a decade later, benefit from significant oil revenues. I will explore the longer-term impact of these additional resources in greater detail later in this chapter, but at the onset of the two reforms, policy-makers in both countries sought to rationalize mental health expenditures by deinstitutionalizing the mentally ill in similar ways. They embraced the same "sectorization" idea developed in France and attempted in the United States.[3] Under this idea, people with mental illness would not usually reside in a hospital; they would receive a comprehensive range of medical outpatient, inpatient, and social care services. To provide these services, governments would assign multidisciplinary teams of mental health professionals to a specific

---

[2] Although the Swedish tax system rendered the counties responsible for financing half of medical care and allowed the municipalities to raise local taxes to support the social services, the degrees of freedom afforded to the localities were small (*Statlig offentlig utredning* 1992:4 Psykiatrin i Norden – ett jämförande perspektiv; hereafter *SOU* 1992:4). Moreover, the Swedish central authorities regulated these powers extensively.

[3] *SOU* 1992:4.

geographic catchment area, rendering them jointly responsible for persons living within that area.

The Swedish/Norwegian divergence in public mental health care is surprising for several other reasons. By their initial similarities and eventual differences, these shadow cases can control for alternative explanations for the divergence in US and French deinstitutionalization trajectories.

Consider first the legacy of state welfare provision. Like France, these Scandinavian societies have a large public sector, which they frequently deploy to provide generous health and social services. In fact, these universalistic, egalitarian, social democratic welfare states are usually even more generous than "conservative" France, which often stratifies benefits by social group (Esping-Andersen 1990). Moreover, the private sector tends to play a more important role in French social welfare, especially its health system, than in Scandinavia. But just as this legacy cannot fully account for the mental health policy outcomes observed in France, neither can it explain those in Scandinavia, for Sweden substantially reduced provision in this area in the 1990s.

Second, consider the question of racial and ethnic diversity, an alternative explanation that emerged in the US case. For most of Sweden and Norway's histories, racial, ethnic, or even religious diversity have not been political flashpoints.[4] Twenty-first-century measures of social fractionalization affirm the perception of cultural homogeneity. According to Alesina and colleagues' influential 2003 index, the probability that two randomly selected individuals belonged to different ethnic groups was just 6 percent in both countries (Alesina et al. 2003).[5] Whether in Norway or Sweden, questions of racial and ethnic diversity have not historically cleaved redistributive politics like in the United States, or even France for that matter (notwithstanding the long-standing importance of their Sámi, Romani, and Finnish-speaking populations, especially in Sweden).

More recently, Norway and Sweden have placed a broadly similar emphasis on multiculturalism and protecting the human rights of international refugees, and this has shaped several waves of immigration in

---

[4] Note also that these histories are partly shared, given the countries' monarchical and diplomatic union of the 19th century. On the significance of historical patterns to the relationship between diversity and public goods provision, see Singh and vom Hau (2016).

[5] This cross-national index, though influential, is imperfect. National census systems, such as those in Scandinavia where data collection on race and ethnicity is limited, may bias its results. Thanks go to Aiysha Varraich for raising this point in personal correspondence in September 2022.

both countries (Brochmann 2018). These groups have included refugees from, for example, the Balkans in the 1990s and the Middle East in the early 2000s. Of the two countries, Sweden has experienced higher rates of migration. Observers of its recent electoral outcomes may wonder if the rise in immigration has reduced social solidarity or increased racial-ethnic animus. Yet scholars emphasize that the political influence of the Radical Right was late and limited in Sweden relative to its Nordic and other West European counterparts (Brochmann 2018). Perhaps as a result, and most notably, Sweden's welfare state appears to be especially inclusive of immigrants (Boräng 2018; Sainsbury 2012). Compared to the United States, Sweden puzzles again. Historically, Sweden did not suffer from the same ethnic, racial, or social fragmentation; nor has its recent rise in immigration fractured its generous welfare state. Yet it too has struggled to provide expansive public mental health services to its population.

Third, the unitary states of Sweden and Norway have enabled both their statist approach to welfare and their national unity. This stands in stark contrast to the United States, where a highly fragmented federal system has made it difficult to develop generous national social policy, including in mental health. The comparison also controls for the possible effect of federalism on policy outcomes. As we will see, the otherwise unitary Sweden did experience a wave of administrative decentralization around the time of the mental health care reforms. Moreover, the country's historic emphasis on local government is conceptually like that of the United States – if not in intensity. Nonetheless, I will discuss this parallel in more detail at the end of the chapter and explore whether and how it may have contributed to policy outcomes in Sweden.

Underpinning the social solidarity of Sweden and Norway, too, are their powerful labor and Left political movements, a fourth alternative explanation that emerges from the French case. But this explanation seems unrelated to mental health care outcomes in Scandinavia, where in fact Sweden's union density (69 percent) is even higher than that of Norway (51 percent) (Kjellberg and Nergaard 2022). Membership rates are more comparable, though also greater, in the public sector: About 70 percent of blue-collar government workers are unionized, as are just over 80 percent among white-collar government workers in both Sweden and Norway (Kjellberg and Nergaard 2022). These workers play an important role in their countries' political economies. Centralized collective bargaining institutions remain anchors of the Swedish and Norwegian economies. Although parts of the industrial relations systems have decentralized for private sector workers, wages for public employees are set at the national level (with some limited local wage-setting in Sweden; Andersen et al. 2015, 148). Moreover, the demands of government employees are often pivotal to national economic negotiations and, increasingly, to party politics. Historically, the Social Democratic party family – Scandinavia's most important – has depended on a powerful labor movement to propel its long-standing success (Hansen 2018, 93). As the public sector has expanded, so too has the Social Democrats' reliance on those employed by it. The usual political-economic influence of the Scandinavian welfare workforce, though, cannot on its own explain the supply of mental health care services, as that of Sweden is now less than that of Norway.

Fifth, the reforms in Sweden and Norway occurred in the 1990s, when the management of public mental health services was no longer as tied to the psychiatric profession as it tended to be in the 1970s and 1980s. In both France and the United States, the public managers that oversaw the mental health reforms in their countries were represented by psychiatric associations. To what extent was their influence a function of their medical, and not managerial, identities? The Swedish–Norwegian comparison controls for this alternative explanation because, by the time of their reforms, the managers of public mental health services were not represented by psychiatric associations. In fact, the Swedish Psychiatric Association has publicly and repeatedly deplored its deliberate exclusion from the reforms, while its Norwegian counterpart has claimed only limited involvement (Åsberg to Sandlund 1989 in Riksarkivet 1/1; SPF 1992; interviews with former presidents of both associations). Public mental health managers instead were represented by the associations of county and municipal governments, also known as the largest "employer" associations in Scandinavia. In Norway, the Norwegian Association of Local and Regional Authorities (Kommunenes Sentralforbund, or KS) represents both county and municipal managers. A similar organization represents these two groups in Sweden as of 2022, but at the time of the reforms they had separate representatives: the Swedish Association of Municipalities (Svenska Kommunförbundet) and the County Council Association (Landstingsförbundet), respectively. This difference was an important one: Although the key managerial representatives in both countries did not double as psychiatric associations, the fragmentation of public managers' representation in Sweden did contribute to the fragmentation of the welfare workforce, as will be shown.

Given that both countries shared these five initial similarities, why is it that their public mental health care systems eventually diverged?

I next examine whether public labor–management coalitions shaped these outcomes. A "method of difference" approach (Mill 1874) allows me to search primarily for the presence or absence of this variable (rather than its mechanistic relationship to the outcome, as in the within-case process analyses of Chapters 4 and 5).

To ensure a comprehensive and parallel survey of the two reforms, I adopt a highly structured empirical strategy, aided by professional translation software and four native Scandinavian-language speakers. We conducted a full review of the secondary literature on Swedish and Norwegian deinstitutionalization, followed by a close reading of the main primary sources that produced each set of reforms: a major governmental report (and any adjacent, minor reports), a set of parliamentary proposals and the subsequent parliamentary debates, and the law that eventually passed. For a guide to these events, see the timelines in Table 6.4.

To understand the role of trade unions, managerial associations, and other interest groups in these reforms, we read the meeting minutes and correspondence of the committee that produced the Swedish government report, as well as the consultation round documents (*remisser*). At the time of writing, these documents were not available for the Norwegian report; so we compensated by interviewing four of its authors and using the "snowball" method to identify two major interest group representatives from the Council for Mental Health (Rådet for psykisk helse; on the method, see Mosley 2013). We also interviewed one author of the Swedish report. Furthermore, we interviewed mental health policy experts in each of the two countries (five in Norway, four in Sweden) and the appropriate heads of the Psychiatric Associations (in Sweden, the president of the Swedish Association at the time of the reform; though, in Norway, only her counterpart's predecessor was available).[6] To redress interviewees' possible memory bias, we corroborated what we learned in interviews with the primary text sources just described, scanned Norwegian and Swedish newspapers for additional information, and then noted in the case studies where this possibility might affect the recounting of events. Last but not least, we engaged in a wide range of informal conversations and email correspondence with colleagues, librarians, archivists, and other experts during four months of field research in Scandinavia.

---

[6] We attempted to contact representatives of labor and management in the two cases, but unfortunately several recent retirements, illnesses, and passings prevented these interviews from occurring (the fieldwork for this chapter was undertaken in 2022, and thus was impacted by the Covid-19 pandemic).

TABLE 6.4 *Timeline of mental health reform process in Sweden and Norway in the 1990s, with main findings*

Event	Sweden	Norway
A government commission issues a report with new policy proposals to deinstitutionalize the mentally ill	1992: Publication of *Statlig offentlig utredning (SOU)* No. 73	1995: Publication of *Norsk offentlig utredning (NOU)* No. 14
Interest groups, including trade unions and personnel representatives, comment on the report in a consultation round and launch advocacy campaigns, which in turn inform the draft proposals to Parliament.	1993: Cabinet drops the proposals that produced disagreement between and across workers and managers at the county and municipal levels in the consultation round.	1996–97: Ministry's draft bill lacks substantial financial commitments. Public sector workers, managers, and other allies in the Council for Mental Health mobilize to advocate for increased investment.
Reform enacted	1995: Parliament passes the Psychiatry Reform to transfer the social care of the mentally ill from the county to municipal levels, with limited funding.	1998–2008: Parliament approves an "Escalation Plan" to expand outpatient and other mental health care services, with ample long-term funding.

NEGATIVE SUPPLY-SIDE POLICY FEEDBACK IN SWEDEN

As in other countries, psychiatric deinstitutionalization had begun in Sweden during the postwar period; but the fiscal strain encountered later in the 20th century prompted the government to speed up the process (Markström 2020; Silfverheim and Steffason 2006). In fact, the cost of care in the large county mental hospitals – many of which could host 1,000 patients – had grown more than any other area of health care in the late 1980s (Lindqvist 2012). These economic realities, combined with the generalized support for outpatient-oriented psychiatry, prompted the then Minister of Health and Social Affairs, Social Democrat Sven Hulterström, to appoint a Commission of Inquiry in 1989. Its task was to evaluate the mental health care system and formally propose new measures to improve its "efficiency" in an "*SOU*" report

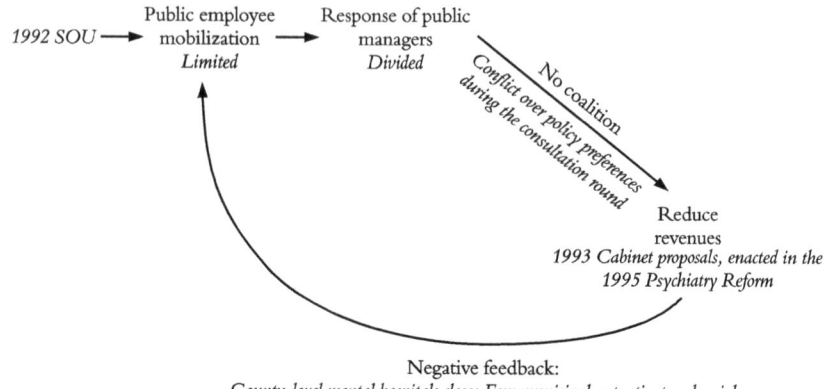

FIGURE 6.3 Negative supply-side policy feedback in Swedish mental health care, 1992–97

(*Statlig offentlig utredning*, or Swedish Government Official Report).[7] This initiative launched the policy-making process that produced the 1995 Psychiatry Reform, with its subsequently negative supply-side policy feedback loop (and ensuing reinforcement over time). This section documents that loop (depicted in Figure 6.3). The absence of a public labor–management coalition first enabled the 1995 Reform and its limited financial support for mental health care (the "feed"), a policy result that in turn further constrained possibilities for workforce advocacy and service expansion (the "back").

I begin by identifying which reforms the Commission proposed in its 1992 *SOU*, how the representatives of the welfare workforce viewed each of them during the consultation period, and what the 1993 right-wing Cabinet subsequently proposed to Parliament. Parliament then passed the proposals with little disagreement and authorized their implementation in 1995. In consensus-oriented Sweden, the responses of interest groups to an Inquiry report directly inform the Cabinet's proposals to Parliament (Petersson 2016). As such, none of the Commission's proposals that produced disagreements between and across labor and management made it to the Cabinet's Propositions. Only one area – where public sector workers and their managers aligned – did. The result was a reform for public mental health care with very limited financial backing.

---

[7] *Statlig offentlig utredning* 1992:73 Välfärd och valfrihet – service, stöd och vård för psykiskt störda; hereafter *SOU* 1992:73.

Consider the results of the three major policy proposals on which managers and workers disagreed. We can begin with the most consequential one: the Commission's proposal to formally devolve social services for the mentally ill to the municipalities. To reduce the number of patients living in mental hospitals at the county level, it proposed decentralizing their "custodial" functions to the municipal level (see Chapter 2 and the Appendix). In theory, the municipalities had received this responsibility more than a decade prior under the 1980 Municipal Social Services Act, but in reality few had developed substantial social services for the mentally ill. The Commission proposed to incentivize municipalities to expand social services over a three-year implementation process: First, municipalities would assume the financial responsibility for patients residing in county mental hospitals for more than six months, with the help of an intragovernmental shift of tax credits. This move would allow the municipalities to develop alternative, nonmedical, and hence less expensive social supports, such that, later, municipalities could assume the financial responsibility for all patients discharged from county mental hospitals (*SOU* 1992:73, 32–33).

Although there was broad consensus about reinforcing the 1980 Municipal Social Services Act, workers and managers at different levels of government disagreed sharply on the specifics of implementation. The six-month residence cut-off was a particularly sensitive flashpoint, in part because of the ideological tension between health professionals and non-health professionals, who argued over whether to require a medical assessment for discharge and whether the cut-off should be shortened to one month.[8]

The question with longer-term consequences was whether the counties should relinquish outpatient mental health services to the municipalities, which in principle only had responsibility over nonmedical social services. If the goal was to deinstitutionalize the mentally ill, municipal-level managers and social care workers argued, they should have "primary responsibility" over the full range of services that would support their lives in the community. Such were the preferences of the Municipal Employers Association (Svenska Kommunförbundet), the Municipal Heads of Social of Services (Foreningen sveriges socialchefer), and the Municipal Employees Union (Sveriges kommunaltjänstemannaförbund,

---

[8] *SOU* 1992:73, 13; Departementspromemoriora 1993:88 *Sammanställning av remissyttranden över Psykiatriutredningens slutbetänkande (SOU 1992:73)*, 97; hereafter Ds 1993:88.

or SKTF). On the other hand, the County Employers' Association (Landstingsförbundet) and county-employed health care staff (such as the Swedish Medical Association) advocated forcefully to retain county control of medical services.[9]

In response, the Cabinet simply reproduced the status quo. Note that both the politicians and civil servants on the Commission seemed to sympathize with the municipalities. In a 1991 letter to the Health Minister, the Commission's parliamentary representative, Bo Holmberg, and a lead civil servant authoring the report, Gert Knuttson, argued that the recent changes to elderly care policy made it possible to task the municipalities with more control over the medical aspects of mental health.[10] Nonetheless, the welfare workforce remained split. Although public labor–management coalitions existed at both the municipal and county level, the two groups stood in opposition to each other. Parliament approved, reinforcing the social service responsibilities of the municipalities and the health service responsibility of the counties.[11] This decision would further exacerbate the fragmentation of the welfare workforce, with consequences for the long-term supply of mental health care.

A second issue was how much money to allocate to the reform, and through which entities. Here the divide was similar to that of the "primary responsibility" debate. The Municipal Employers Association, the Municipal Heads of Social Services, and the Municipal Employees Union (SKTF) advocated for additional financial support to municipal social services, while the County Employers' Association and medical staff advocated for more financing at the county level (*SOU* 1992:73, 495–510; Ds 1993:88, chap. 9). Note that some workers raised concerns about this fragmentation. The SKTF, in a strongly worded letter to the Ministry of Social Affairs, warned about carrying out the reform "with totally inadequate resources and without adequate planning and cooperation between administrators and the various staff groups concerned" (Sture to Petterson in Riksarkivet 1/4). But such warnings would have little effect on public policy.

---

[9] Swedish law forbids municipalities from employing physicians. Historically, the Swedish Medical Association has defended this statute in order to preserve professional unity, as employees of a single level of government (personal communication with Stig Montin, July 2022). Also, note both here in the Swedish case and next in the Norwegian case that private sector providers are absent from reform discussions. This artifact of the social democratic welfare tradition stands in contrast to the American and French contexts, where private medical practice has been more common.

[10] Riksarkivet 1/3; for the policy changes, see Proposition 1990/1991:14 *Om ansvaret för service och vård till äldre och handikappade m. m*; hereafter Prop 1990/91:14.

[11] Proposition 1993/1994:218 *Psykiskt stördas villkor*; hereafter Prop 1993/94: 218.

Noting these conflicts and the emergence of similar ones in other decentralizing policy areas, the Cabinet instead opted to delay their resolution, setting up a parliamentary committee to "find a solution with broad support in the world of local government" (referring to both counties and municipalities; Prop 1993/94: 218, sec. 6.5). Setting aside the structural fiscal questions that would increase funding to either counties or municipalities (or both), the government instead offered a short-term implementation grant of 1.2 billion SEK (or about $200 million contemporary USD), to be paid between 1995 and 1997 (Prop 1993/94: 218, 3). That limited funding would soon make it difficult to expand and develop mental health care.

In a third controversial proposal, the Commission sought to grant people with mental illnesses the legal right to demand services from counties and municipalities by attaching that right to a recent bill passed for people with physical disabilities, the 1992 "*LSS*."[12] Here the positions of public managers, at both county and municipal levels, differed from the health and social care unions that represented their employees. The Municipal Employers Association, the Municipal Heads of Social of Services, and the County Employers Association worried that the "increased social costs" and "economic effects" would be too high if the mentally ill gained this right (Ds 1993:88, 50). Indeed, if the administrative court ruled in a mentally ill person's favor, counties and municipalities would be legally obligated to provide them with the requested services. Meanwhile, workers (including the Swedish Medical Association) generally supported the Commission's proposal; the demands of the mentally ill would likely expand their opportunities for work (Ds 1993:88, 52, 36). Unions that represented blue-collar and social workers, those most likely to benefit from this policy change, even favored expanding the benefits' eligibility rules to broaden the scope of potential clients (see LO and SKAF comments in Ds 1993:88, 52). Taking explicit note of these divisions (Prop 1993/94: 218, sec. 5.3–4), the Cabinet took what Urban Markström refers to as a "wait-and-see" approach (Markström 2003, chap. 6). Leveraging rifts in the welfare workforce to avoid public spending increases, the Cabinet claimed it needed "more accurate information on the scope of the law and its financial implications" (Prop 1993/94: 218, 28). As a result, the mentally ill did not gain the legal right to demand services in 1995.

---

[12] Prop 1992/1993:159 *Lag om stöd och service till vissa funktionshindrade*; hereafter Prop 1992/93:159 or simply *LSS*.

Managers and workers, though, did agree on something: "personal assistants." The broad support for trialing this new occupational group provides a useful counterfactual. The Cabinet indeed was willing to allocate resources to policies jointly supported by both managers and workers. A concept inspired by the Anglo-American case worker, the personal assistant would offer individualized support to persons with mental illness. That some observers critiqued the idea as a foreign import seemed to make little difference to the welfare workforce (Maycraft Kall 2010; Ds 1993:88, 58). If enacted with financial support, the personal assistants' scheme could bring new members to the unions and new funds to employers. The details were vague. Workers and managers wondered about the skill level, legal status, and of course appropriate employer of the personal assistant. In principle the assistants would be employed at the municipal level, though several unions were quick to note that workers at both levels of government, such as county-employed allied health professionals or nurses, could take on this new role as well (Ds 1993:88, 52). The potential flexibility of the personal assistant may have been its selling point to a broad spectrum of workers and managers across levels of government. Responding in the affirmative to their united stance, the government proposition enacted the scheme with a three-year trial period and its own, separate funding to "stimulate [the program's] development" (Prop 1993/94: 218, sec. 5.3). Furthermore, according to a lead author of the *SOU*, "the government actually gave more money than we could think of!" Not only did politicians concede to reforms supported by both workers and managers, but it also seems that they did so generously.[13]

Overall, however, the fragmentation of the welfare workforce allowed the 1995 Reform to both restrict the funds available for mental health care expansion and exacerbate existing political divisions. As a result, negative returns to services and the workforce played out over the next decades (part two of the feedback loop). In fact, studies of the 1995 Reform's implementation suggest that it was difficult for the welfare workforce to unite in favor of expanding services. Among the greatest challenges was that managers and workers could not plan ahead: The temporary grant program provided no long-term funding guarantees, rendering it difficult

---

[13] Note also that a couple of key Cabinet members had been especially supportive of the personal assistants' policy during the passage of the 1992 *LSS*, a factor that may have helped to boost their funding allocation in the 1995 Psychiatry Reform (personal communication with Carl Dahlström, drawing on research conducted for Dahlström 2009).

to hire new personnel or establish a durable operations program. When funding limitations resulted in staff cuts, furthermore, quality of care suffered (see Tidemalm's 1996 and 2000 studies of a group housing program in Markström 2003, chap. 7). The lack of financial security in this policy area thus facilitated those cuts and offered managers and workers few opportunities to redress them.

Not only were workers bereft of generous and secure funding; it also became more challenging to identify to whom they should express their grievances. Confusion was especially rife at the municipal level, since the Reform provided very little guidance on how to develop new social services for the mentally ill, an approach that Wendy Maycraft Kall's (2010) study referred to as central government's "soft steering" of local policy. As a result, municipalities developed a myriad of approaches to organizing services for the mentally ill. The "managers" of these services, Markström (2003, chap. 8) found, could range from the Municipal Head of Social Services, to a "psychiatric coordinator," to the director of a service primarily targeted at another client group (such as those with physical impairments). That the political representation of each of these administrators varied, moreover, made it even more difficult for unions to identify potential coalition partners.[14] Sentiments like this one, uttered by one of his interviewees, aptly captures the confusion of workers: "They have an awful lot of managers ... in social services: middle managers and assistant managers and coordinators. It seems to be difficult, you don't know which manager to go to and who does what" (staff member at a residence support group for people with mental illness, Markström 2003, chap. 8, 12). The Reform's soft steering contributed to the increasing fragmentation and complexity of the management hierarchy, obscuring the coalition possibilities for workers. Moreover, the limited agitation from workers appears to have contributed to what Markström (2003, chap. 8) called managers' overall "passive" approach to the Reform's implementation. They had little incentive to take up the funds and expand services.

[14] As of 2022, the political representatives of public psychiatric managers in Sweden could be represented by the County and Municipal Employers Association (Sveriges Kommuner och Regioner), the Municipal Heads of Social of Services, the Municipal Employees Union, or trade unions and associations unions representing nurses, psychologists, psychiatrists, or other professional leadership. None of these organizations, furthermore, represents solely psychiatric managers, and as such they must balance the demands of those managers with those of their other members. The same is true of mental health and social care employees, who are spread between, for example, nurses' unions, social workers' unions, the SKTF, Kommunal, and medical associations.

More generally, the Reform deepened the divide between county-level employers and health workers on the one hand and municipal-level employers and social care workers on the other. Disagreements about whether and how much to allocate to each level of government for the care of the mentally ill continued in the years following its enactment. County-level medical staff have little in common with municipal-level social care staff. What is more, there is a sharp professional divide. Consider what occurred when county-level mental hospitals closed and transferred some former staff to municipal social service employment (often against their will). Numerous studies documented how these workers felt out of place, even devalued, in their new positions and had difficulty finding common ground with employees of other social care institutions (see Johansson and Westin 1997 cited in Markström 2003, chap. 7). The de-professionalization of parts of the psychiatric workforce, furthermore, may have weakened the workforce's political strength. This will stand in sharp contrast with the Norwegian approach discussed in the next section, where significant upskilling took place. Indeed, by de-professionalizing and fragmenting the Swedish welfare workforce, no coalition could successfully advocate for more funding for mental health care from Parliament, reinforcing the negative feedback loop (see Figure 6.3).

Nonetheless, it is worth noting the few local examples where services did expand: In areas where mental health care workers were powerful, managers were keen to ally with them, and the coalition could depend on alternative, and more secure, funding streams. Indeed, the most "ambitious" municipalities tended to be "mental hospital towns," that is, towns where psychiatric services, and by extension staff, were already present (Markström 2003, chap. 2; Markström and Lindqvist 2015). One can infer that the high density of psychiatric employees would have increased the political pressure to expand services in these municipalities after the Reform. Markström (2003) also found ample evidence that the coordination and coalition-building efforts of local management (across both county-level health care and municipal-level social services) contributed to service expansion as well. Due to the ample structural and organizational setbacks in the area, though, these "moral entrepreneurs" often built these coalitions out of sheer goodwill rather than personal self-interest (Markström 2019; 2003, chap. 2).

The services best suited to expansion, moreover, were those that could draw on other, more secure financing streams and fewer staff, such as sheltered housing units, or those that had obtained financial support due to an alliance between managers and workers in the first place, such as the personal assistants' scheme (Markström 2003). Even still, only about 60 sheltered housing projects were launched in Sweden as a result of the Reform (in fact the stimulus grant was never even fully used) and the personal assistants' scheme has experienced only limited growth (Markström 2003, chaps. 7–8).

POSITIVE SUPPLY-SIDE POLICY FEEDBACK IN NORWAY

From one standpoint, the genesis of the Norwegian mental health reforms is virtually identical to that of Sweden: A 1995 *NOU* report (*Norsk offentlig utredning*, or Norwegian Government Official Report) evaluated the expensive, county-based long-term care system and proposed new policies aimed at reorienting the system toward community-based outpatient and social care services with the help of municipal governments.[15] Although the *NOU* included a review of care for the elderly and disabled, significant attention was also paid to the mentally ill. To accommodate the overflow of patients in mental hospitals, Norway had established the aforementioned "psychiatric nursing homes" in the 1970s to house patients with severe and chronic mental illness over the long term, such that by 1990 these institutions had become de facto asylums. The *NOU* hence proposed repurposing these institutions as outpatient-oriented services, namely "district psychiatry centers," a concept in fact inspired by the US community mental health centers (*NOU* 1995: 14, 58–60; interview with the Norwegian civil servant responsible for overseeing mental health financing at the time of the reform).

On the other hand, the strength and unity of the welfare workforce prior to the 1995 *NOU* report presents a strong contrast to the case of Sweden. Potent advocacy from public sector workers, managers, and their allies was already underway well before the 1995 report went to press. In 1992, the Norwegian public broadcaster NRK (Norsk rikskringkasting) selected the Council for Mental Health – an advocacy group composed of representatives from numerous organizations, including trade unions and professional associations – as its partner in its annual fundraising telethon, TV-aksjonen. Known as the world's

---

[15] Compared to the *SOU*, the *NOU* did propose a longer residential cut-off. The Norwegian report suggested transferring psychiatric patients out of the county long-term care institutions after twelve months of residency, not six (or one), as in Sweden. *Norsk offentlig utredning* 1995:14 Fylkeskommunale langtidsinstitusjoner; hereafter *NOU* 1995:14.

largest fundraising campaign, Norway's telethon highlights the work of a chosen nongovernmental organization while collecting voluntary public donations for the cause. Although the Council had begun as a research organization in 1985, it drew on the 90 million NOK (over $20 million contemporary USD; per Norges Bank 2023b; OECD 2023) collected from the 1992 civic campaign to complete its transformation into a political lobby. Over the following years, the Council and its members held conferences throughout the country to raise awareness of mental health issues. Crucially, these conferences brought together mental health professionals, their trade union representatives, local administrators and managers, as well as patients and parliamentarians. The combination was potent. Patient stories drew heavy media coverage, while members of Parliament developed closer ties and commitments to the mental health care workforce in their local districts. The Council had thrown mental health into the spotlight while rendering electorally minded politicians accountable to this policy area.[16]

These two factors came together in 1995, producing the first part of a positive supply-side policy feedback loop (see Figure 6.4). The Council – by then, well-resourced both financially and politically – sprang into action upon the *NOU*'s publication. Its unity was its greatest strength. Although its members did not always agree on policy, the Council required the internal resolution of these debates before expressing a shared preference to the authorities. In the words of its former Secretary General, this protocol allowed the group to have a "clearer and more precise influence" on the reform process.

The same quote could describe the organization representing both municipalities and county administrators (KS). In contrast to their counterparts in Sweden, managers at both these levels of government organized together. This organizational structure promoted the joint expression of policy preferences and headed off any fragmentation. Note also that the KS did not formally join the Council for Mental Health. In some ways, the relationship between the KS and the Council resembled that of traditional industrial relations, with managers (KS) on the

---

[16] Interview with former Chair of the Council for Mental Health; see also "90 millioner til psykisk helse," *Aura Avis.* May 29, 1993; "Krever mer til psykisk helse," *Arbeiderbladet.* September 15, 1995; "Samler inn psykiatri-underskrifter," *Harstad Tidende.* September 29, 1995; "Vellykket TV-aksjon: 90 millioner til psykisk helse," *Indre Smaalenenes Avis.* May 28, 1993; "Verdensdag for psykisk helsevern," *Nationen.* October 4, 1994; Elisabeth Vogt, "50 pasienter kan miste behandlingstilbudet," *Moss Avis*, October 9, 1995.

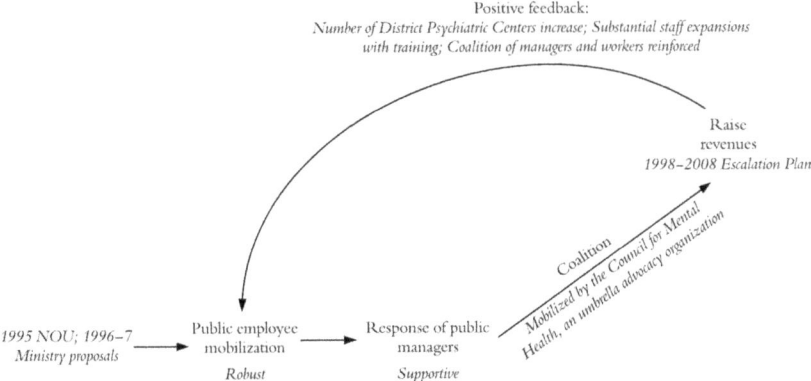

FIGURE 6.4 Positive supply-side policy feedback in Norwegian mental health care, 1995–2008

one side and workers (the Council) on the other side of the negotiating table.[17] Because only one organization spoke for each end (all public managers and all their employees, respectively), agreements between them were universally beneficial to public employees across all levels of government and types of occupations.

When the Ministry published its proposals to Parliament in 1996–7, the Council continued its pressure, particularly regarding the need for funding, a question that the Ministry had effectively ignored.[18] Although Norway's financial crisis was less severe than Sweden's at the time, its bureaucrats were no more keen to devote significant resources to the reform. The proposals, while in line with the joint preferences of managers and workers, lacked substantial financial commitments. In fact, at the press conference announcing the reform proposals, the then Chair of the Council exclaimed, "But where is the money?!" – a pointed line that has become among the most memorable and repeated by those in attendance.[19] In response, the Council, its members, and allies in the Ministry undertook a second round of intensive advocacy. Another tour

---

[17] Of course, their relationship was not one of formal collective bargaining, especially since the Council also aimed to speak for those not employed by the mental health system, such as academic researchers and patients.

[18] Stortingsmelding 1996–1997: 25 Åpenhet og helhet: Om psykiske lidelser og tjenestetilbudene; hereafter 1996–97 St meld 25.

[19] Former Chair of the Council for Mental Health, interview with the author, August 2022; Three Norwegian civil servants (Lead author of the 1995 *NOU* Report; Assistant Director of the Board of Health; and Deputy Minister of Health), joint interview with the author, July 2022.

of conferences around the country, combined with active parliamentary lobbying, pressured politicians to both accept the proposals and commit considerable funds to them. "This is the most discussed [Ministerial proposal] ever," its lead author purportedly exclaimed (interview with former Chair of the Council for Mental Health).

The coalition produced astounding results. The proposals for the usually small and politically insignificant issue of mental health care reform gained unanimous support in Parliament, which publicly commended "the Council for Mental Health and its important work" in the enactment process.[20] Moreover, the conservative Parliament berated the Ministry for not providing enough funds in its original proposal and pressed for redress:

The [Parliament's Social Welfare] Committee believes that increased earmarked funding for mental health care will be necessary for many years to come ... [and] would like to point out that the [Ministry's proposal] does not contain calculations and figures that can give a sufficient basis for estimating how much money to allocate to psychiatry in the coming years ... A major effort must now be made for people with mental disorders ... The Committee requests that a binding action plan for psychiatry be prepared that includes ... a financially binding escalation plan for the earmarked subsidy.[21]

With this strong and urgent language, the politicians moved to earmark a whopping 24 billion NOK (about $5 billion contemporary USD) for the project to spend over the following eight years.[22] Counties would decrease the resident populations of their long-term mental health care institutions while both counties and municipalities would increase the provision of community-based alternatives. While municipalities gained significant financial support to expand social services (like their counterparts in Sweden, though with far more funding), Norwegian counties also gained financially; they would implement the district psychiatry centers. The earmarked funds also supported the hiring and upskilling of personnel. This move gave trade unions a pipeline of potential new members and even direct financial support, for they often administered the new training programs (interview with Norwegian civil servant mental health financing expert).

---

[20] "Psykiske lidelser og tjenestetilbudene," *Stortingstidende* June 17, 1997, 4274; for the votes, 4311–12.

[21] Innstilling fra sosialkomiteen om psykiske lidelser og tjenestetilbudene (Åpenhet og helhet) 1996–1997: 258, sec. 8.2; hereafter 1996–97 Innst. S. 258.

[22] Proposisjon til Stortinget 1997–1998: 63 *Om opptrappingsplan for psykisk helse 1999–2006, Endringer i statsbudsjettet for 1998.*

The result was the positive second part of the feedback loop (see Figure 6.4). The presence of a robust public labor–management coalition helped to ensure the implementation of the "Escalation Plan" over the following decade (the coalition also managed to extend the project by two years). Counties, municipalities, and their employees only received financing for service expansion if and when they submitted an implementation plan, which included the requisite set of services and staff. Although some managers complained about these firm requirements, in general the mental health workforce was keen to accept the new earmarked funds.[23] Moreover, the Council for Mental Health and its allies acted as implementation watchdogs. As the Council's former Secretary General put it, the organization would "highlight whether the authorities actually granted what they were supposed to and whether the municipalities actually used the earmarked funds for what they were required to do."[24] Of particular note was the Council's advocacy for the expansion of new mental health resources and positions. Although some municipalities preferred to simply convert pre-existing health and social care facilities and staff into resources for the mental health sector, the Council instead advocated for more facilities and more staff.

The result of this coalition and the policy feedback loop it facilitated was the production of the policy outcomes in Table 6.1. Even as psychiatric nursing homes were downsized, the number of district psychiatry centers increased, as did their staff. By the end of the Escalation Plan, supply-side policy feedback had increased total staffing in mental health by 20 percent (Romøren 2018). The positive feedback, furthermore, appears to have continued. Norwegian public policy stipulates that the State must spend more on mental health care than somatic care, and as of 2023 a new Escalation Plan is underway at the Ministry.[25]

---

[23] Indeed, earmarking was at first an issue where managers and workers could not agree. Managers wanted more flexibility on the use of funds than workers. But the Council for Mental Health, which represented staff employed specifically in psychiatry, heavily pressured the managers' organization, KS, to accept earmarking; and it succeeded (interview with the former Secretary General of the Council for Mental Health).

[24] Ibid.

[25] Helse- og omsorgsdepartementet, "Opptrappingsplan for psykisk helse," *Press Room, Regjeringen.no*, April 4, 2022, www.regjeringen.no/no/aktuelt/opptrappingsplan-psykisk-helse/id2907606/; Stortingsmelding 2023–2023: 23 Opptrappingsplan for psykisk helse (2023–2033).

DISCUSSION AND CONCLUSION

The absence of consensus between (and across) public sector managers and workers in Swedish mental health care facilitated negative supply-side policy feedback during the 1990s. In contrast, a forceful, formally organized coalition enabled positive supply-side policy feedback in Norwegian mental health care. In each case, I have traced a single loop launched in the 1990s, in contrast to the previous chapters on the United States and France, where three respective feedback cycles gradually reinforced contrasting patterns of deinstitutionalization. The results of the 1990s may have positioned Swedish and Norwegian mental health care policy and staff to experience several more self-reinforcing feedback cycles in the future as well, though the argument of this book does not aim to be deterministic. Theoretically, a coalition of managers and workers could emerge in Sweden and disappear in Norway. Nonetheless, contemporary levels of mental health care supply in the two countries (as well as the political momentum behind launching a second Escalation Plan in Norway) suggest a pattern of continued reinforcement since the 1990s, such that their diverging policy results have endured.

Although these two countries share much in common, readers familiar with their differences might wonder about whether and how three of these differences could have shaped these politics. To conclude this chapter, I consider whether and how contemporaneous differences between Sweden and Norway's economic crises and right-wing governments may have shaped mental health care reform in either case. I also examine the effect of Sweden's greater emphasis on decentralization. To be sure, this shadow "most similar systems" comparison does not allow for a fine-grained assessment of case-specific alternative hypotheses; but it is nonetheless important to briefly consider a few pertinent questions.

First, and perhaps most importantly, did Sweden's deeper economic downturns render retrenchment more likely than in Norway? Conversely, did Norway's access to oil revenues over-determine the expansion of public mental health services in that country? Although both countries experienced banking crises in the 1990s, between 1990 and 1993 average loss provisions amounted to 4.8 percent in Sweden, compared to 2.7 percent in Norway (Honkapohja 2009, 10). Not only did Sweden face greater financial pain but it also commenced its reforms precisely at that time. Norway, on the other hand, waited until the worst of the downturn had passed to reform (and expand) public mental health care. Moreover, the growth rate of the Norwegian oil fund escalated significantly in the following decade, as the Escalation Plan was underway. Technical quibbles notwithstanding (Norway's recovery was slow, and in fact current accounts had fallen when the Escalation Plan passed), fiscal pressures were objectively greater in Sweden than in Norway at the onset of the reform. Later, during implementation, Norway would benefit from a wellspring of funds.

Recall that in Norway, however, the Ministry's civil servants did not make financial requests of Parliament in their original proposal (1996–97 St meld 25). Yet elected politicians ultimately allocated a conspicuous amount of funding – far beyond what might have been expected at the time – to implementation (1996–97 Innst. S. 258; 1997–98 St prp 63). What occurred between these two steps? As any observer of economic inequality would note, politicians in resource-rich countries do not always choose to distribute that wealth to the needy. As the case study illustrates, the advocacy of the Council for Mental Health and its welfare workforce membership proved essential for motivating politicians to increase the size of those allocations. Had a consensus between managers and workers not existed in Norway, politicians may have been just as likely to use the economic crisis as an excuse to restrict their financial support for the reforms. Instead, they catapulted funding in this area. Certainly, after the reform passed, Norway's increasing wealth helped to boost the funds available for the Escalation Plan, which no doubt helped to justify its two-year extension. But it is important to remember that politicians committed resources to mental health care before this windfall occurred.

Moreover, Sweden did devote significant resources to other social policy areas at this time. Major reforms to both the elderly care system and the disability care system occurred just before the mental health care reform, amounting to 5.5 billion and 1.6 billion SEK respectively (over $1 billion and about $300 million contemporary USD; Prop 1990/91:14 and Prop 1992/93:159; per OECD 2023; SCB 2023). The budgets allocated to these changes were much higher, perhaps in part because of their different constituencies. As in other countries, the interest groups representing older adults and people with physical disabilities tend to be more politically influential than those that represent people with mental disabilities, whose condition makes it especially difficult to mobilize. In addition, middle-class families are more likely to demand caregiving support for their older parents and, if to a lesser extent, relatives with physical disabilities than for their comparatively fewer relatives with severe psychiatric needs. Sweden allocated more funding to reforms in these two other areas than in mental health, both during the crisis and after it. Even as the economy picked up again in the late 1990s, far fewer resources were distributed to mental health care than to elderly care or disability support. By then, the negative feedback loop in mental health care had established itself in ways that continued to weaken this sector relative to other social policy areas.

If one steps back to compare the financial commitments in both cases, furthermore, the sheer magnitude of the difference in scale between them stands out (Table 6.1). In effect, Norway committed to spending over tenfold more per capita per year than Sweden, and for four times as long. These outcomes are strikingly divergent: Sweden spent far less than one might expect from a country with generous public service provision and Norway spent far more on a policy area that rarely receives substantial financial resources. It is difficult to explain these differences without attending to the politics that produced them.

A second alternative explanation accordingly considers the effects of political partisanship: Did the right-wing government and policy priorities of early 1990s Sweden bias outcomes in that country? The general elections of 1991 had dealt a serious blow to the long-standing dominance of the Social Democrats, generating a liberal-conservative Cabinet committed to fiscal restraint and marketization. The Cabinet sought to introduce these changes to a range of social welfare and public service areas, notably including care for the elderly and disabled. In some ways, the reforms in mental health care aligned well with these aims (even though the Ädel reforms may have received more financial and political attention).

The government that passed the Norwegian Escalation Plan was also a government of the Right, but of a very different character than Sweden's at that time. The Norwegian elections of 1997 had brought Christian Democrats to power. Although this family of parties may prefer limited government, Christian Democrats stand out for their historic sympathies for the poor and marginalized (van Kersbergen 1995). As Rogers (2022) has found, these sympathies extend to the mentally ill as well. Moreover, Norway's Christian Democratic prime minister, Kjell Magne Bondevik, personally experienced and publicly acknowledged mental illness, so much so that in 1998 he took time away from office to recover from a depressive episode. One must nevertheless ask whether the Norwegian Christian Democrats would have allocated quite so much financial support to mental health care absent the advocacy of the public labor–management coalition.[26] This political party typically prefers to deliver social services through nongovernment, church, and family institutions, rather than the state (van Kersbergen 1995). More broadly, the reforms were timed with overall right-wing partisanship, a variable that cross-national studies associate with cuts, not expansions, to social spending (e.g., Huber and Stephens 2000).

Third, what role does decentralization play? Norway's more centralized polity, for instance, appears to have helped unite its welfare workforce. Although both countries have unitary states, Sweden's historic emphasis on local self-government – and its rise in the 1990s – renders public policy there somewhat less centralized than in Norway (Laegrid 2018). This difference appears to have fragmented Sweden's public sector workforce in the 1990s, contributing to the negative supply-side policy feedback process. A closer look at the impact of decentralization in Sweden and (more) centralization in Norway underscores several theoretical points discussed in Chapter 1.

It underscores the importance of management qua management to supply-side policy feedback, even if (or especially because) the substantive content of managerial divisions can vary. Like their counterparts in the previous chapters on the United States and France, public sector managers in Sweden sought to clearly demarcate and protect their administrative territory. What is more, the fierce debates between municipal and county managers over who had "primary responsibility" over mental health care show that managerial divisions can appear within the public sector, not just between the public and private sectors. Unlike their counterparts in the previous chapters, however, public managers in Sweden did not seek to protect medical territory. They were not physicians. In fact, the administrative goals of psychiatrists were all but ignored (SPF 1992, sec. 4.2.2). Rather, the Swedish case demonstrates how public sector managers influence policy even without a medical degree, and in what ways they too can practice ring-fencing within the public sector itself. In brief, managers matter to supply-side policy feedback because they are managers, not because they are doctors wielding medical authority.

It underscores, furthermore, the importance of organizational form. While county and municipal managers organized together in Norway,

---

[26] Worth noting as well is that both countries adopted "New Public Management" in approaches in the 1990s (Laegrid 2018; see also Romøren 2018). These public administration reforms drew on private sector concepts and strategies, sometimes producing fewer, or otherwise more marketized, public services as a result.

they did not in Sweden until later (they have since joined forces). As in the French and American cases, different organizational forms produce different vehicles for preference expression, with different results. Forced to speak with one political voice, county and municipal managers in Norway likely came to agreement in ways not politically feasible for their Swedish counterparts. The same could be said of Norwegian workers employed by different levels of government and in different services, as their joint participation in the Council for Mental Health also facilitated consensus.[27]

As such, it underscores that workers can also be divided, reinforcing divisions among public sector managers and producing multiple, ineffective public labor–management coalitions. Since counties employ health care workers and municipalities employ social care workers, the welfare workforce split along sectoral lines in two out of the four policy issues studied. The fact that county-level workers were higher-skill and physicians could not work at the municipal level only cemented this divide further. As a result, there were in fact two public labor–management coalitions over these issues (between social care workers and municipal managers and between health care staff and county managers). Neither coalition, though, was successful. A conventional labor–management split followed in the third issue; that too was unsuccessful. For positive supply-side policy feedback to take off, it seems, a single coalition of public managers and workers must be present, as was the case in the fourth policy issue.

Lastly, it underscores that institutional factors can shape the possibilities for coalition, though that cause need not be intentional nor its effect definitive. Sweden's long tradition of local government notwithstanding, the government had only recently begun to decentralize in earnest. This changing and often foggy landscape both weakened incentives and challenged the efforts of workers and managers at county and municipal levels of government to coordinate. It is not evident that the state intended to fragment the welfare workforce in this way. Such a claim would require a more precise definition of the state and who within it had the (rare) foresight to carry out this plan. Just as important, however, is the fact that structural factors do not unequivocally determine coalitional possibilities. The mobilization efforts of the Council for Mental Health

---

[27] Unfortunately, I cannot describe how municipal and county interests came to agreement within each of these organizations. Meeting minutes and other internal documents of the KS and the Council for Mental Health were unavailable during the fieldwork period.

in Norway or the occasional local examples that emerged in Sweden, for instance, show the importance of human agency in producing the outcomes observed there. The alternative explanation of administrative decentralization, then, both complements and clarifies the primary argument presented in this book.

In conclusion, a shadow comparison of the contrasting public mental health care reforms in Sweden and Norway in the 1990s is supportive of my hypothesis. Despite the many similarities between the two countries, Sweden and Norway took opposite approaches when they formalized their deinstitutionalization policies, such that the supply of public mental health care decreased in Sweden and increased in Norway. A review of both primary and secondary sources points to a core difference between the two countries: the political alliances and strategies of the welfare workforce. Where public sector managers and workers in Sweden could not come to agreement on how to reform the mental health care system, unifying organizations in Norway brought them to consensus and amplified their advocacy efforts. The result was, as hypothesized, negative and positive supply-side policy feedback, respectively.

Feedback processes such as these, moreover, can shape policies far beyond those in mental health. In the following and final chapter of this book, I explore the implications of these findings for the welfare state, other public services, and indeed the macroeconomy as a whole. In so doing, it focuses on three key trends: the welfare state's emphatic shift from cash transfers in the postwar period to social services in the late 20th century; the rise of public service employment, now a linchpin of the advanced economies; and a new distributional logic of welfare provision. Increasingly, it is public sector – not private sector – unions that shape social policy. The politics of psychiatric deinstitutionalization therefore offer a window into these trends, illuminating several key dimensions and raising questions for future research.

7

Beyond Deinstitutionalization

Welfare Workers and Welfare Capitalism

Much of this book has focused on the 20th century, when public employees played a crucial role in developing contemporary mental health care systems. But the political, economic, and social relevance of the "welfare workforce" is far from a historical curiosity.[1] In just the first decade of the 21st century, employment in health and social services accounted for more than a quarter of employment growth in high-income economies (European Commission 2010). Moreover, this trend did not reverse during the 2008 economic crisis, when employment decreased in other sectors (European Commission 2014). Since then, public employment has continued to expand, with consequences for the politics of the welfare state.

After reviewing my core findings about psychiatric deinstitutionalization and mental health care, in this concluding chapter I lay out my argument's theoretical implications for social policy scholarship more generally. It highlights that the political logic of social services, which now account for almost half of welfare state programs, is distinct from that of cash transfers (e.g., pensions, unemployment, disability benefits). The key difference: the welfare workforce. These actors are driving social service infrastructure in ways underexplored and underappreciated by existing scholarship. The policy implications of this trend, moreover, are complex, especially as the contours of the welfare workforce become less clear. I close by considering how to harness the power of welfare workers in contemporary welfare capitalism.

---

[1] As discussed, this term refers to those who depend on the welfare state for their employment, such as nurses, teachers, caregivers, facility support staff, and, importantly, supervisors.

CORE FINDINGS ABOUT DEINSTITUTIONALIZATION
AND MENTAL HEALTH CARE

I began this book with a simple observation: Not all western countries deinstitutionalized psychiatric patients in the same way. Although similar factors prompted these societies to reduce the proportion of their population residing in mental hospitals, only some governments subsequently closed those institutions. Such was the case of the archetypical examples of the United States and the United Kingdom. In some countries, however, deinstitutionalization did not result in the wholesale closure of mental hospitals (e.g., France, Norway). In fact, some societies deinstitutionalized by expanding both hospital and non-hospital mental health care (Figure 7.1). Correlated with these outcomes is heavy public investment, a factor that not only renders the mental health care market distinct from the general health care market but also helps to explain the significant role of public sector trade unions in its politics.

Indeed, the observed variation in patterns of deinstitutionalization and mental health care has been driven by public sector employees, that is,

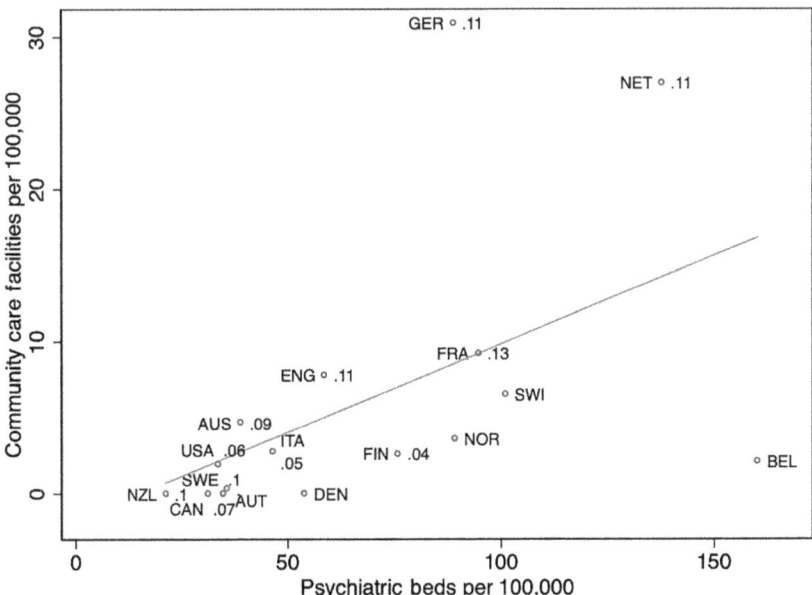

FIGURE 7.1 Scatterplot of psychiatric beds and community care facilities per 100,000 in 16 high-income democracies, with percentage of health budget allocated to mental health (as available) and line of best fit
Source: WHO (2011)

those who have depended on these services for their employment. Mental health policy thus offers a window into the political economy of services for vulnerable populations. Programs whose recipients lack political, economic, and social resources tend to gain little support (van Oorschot et al. 2017; Weir et al. 1988). Absent a powerful client interest group, the maintenance and expansion of public services can depend on those who rely on them for their employment: Public employees can advocate for service provision when their clients cannot. This is precisely what occurred in mental health, where the advocacy of public employees helped to expand services in some countries, despite broader deinstitutionalization trends.

The preceding chapters have documented how the mobilization of public employees to raise their wages and protect their employment can produce powerful "policy feedback" effects (Figure 7.2), with the result of shoring up the provision of mental health care and other services for marginalized populations. Similar to those self-reinforcing (or self-undermining) policy–client relationships documented at the mass level (e.g., Campbell 2003; Mettler 2005; Soss 1999) and the elite level (e.g., Patashnik 2008; Pierson 1996; Weir and Skocpol 1985), this meso-level version of policy feedback links policies and public servants. If the welfare workforce achieves its aims, new or expanded resources can empower it further, spurring additional rounds of "supply-side" policy feedback and client service provision. Whether public employees succeed, however, depends on their degree of political influence. Although a wide range of conditions can shape this influence, I emphasized the role of political allies, in particular, their managers.

The public labor–management coalition is a distinctive source of public employee power, as workers and managers in that sector often share more common interests than their counterparts in the private sector. But what might explain, then, the presence or absence of such a special alliance? It is the independent and unified representation of public managers. The findings presented here confirm that when public managers can express their interests together and independently of private managers, they are more likely to form a coalition with public sector workers. The mechanisms of "brokerage" and "adaptive expectations" then come into play: Managers draw on the various levers at their disposal to influence policy-makers, who in turn concede to their demands in order to avoid escalating retribution from the powerful coalition. But if public sector supervisors organize with private sector supervisors or if the representation of public sector managers is split among multiple organizations, then their shared representatives must contend with the different positions of

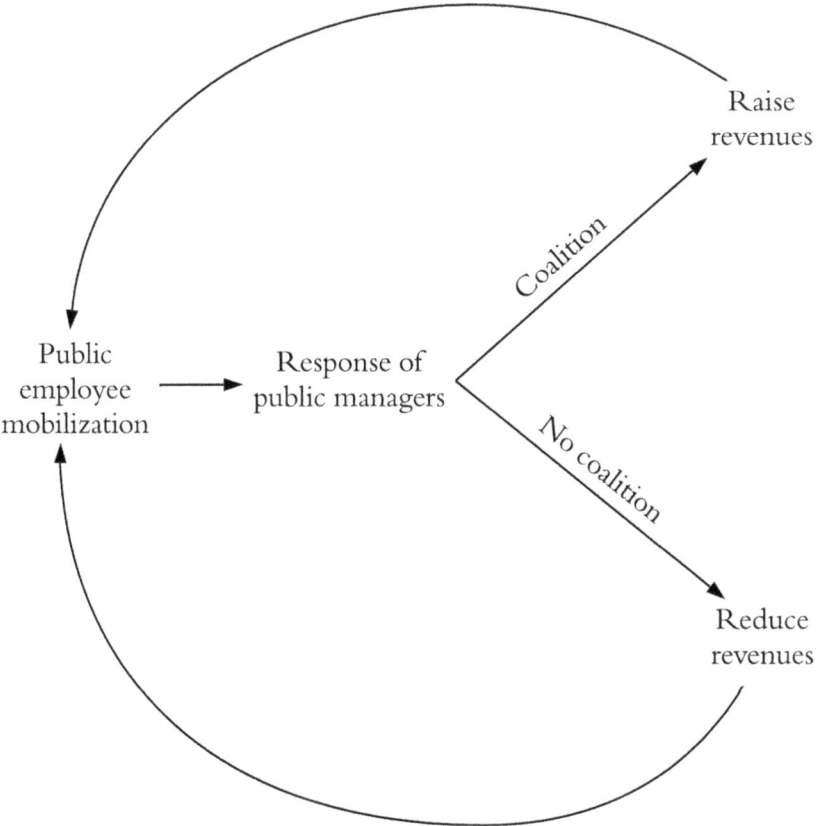

Positive feedback:
more public services, employment security and
protections, workforce growth, support for labor rights

Negative feedback:
fewer public services, reduced wages and
protections, layoffs, less support for labor rights

FIGURE 7.2 Supply-side policy feedback model: Effects of public sector worker alliances on the supply of public social services for disenfranchised populations (basic diagram of theoretical argument)

each camp. This means that their representatives must make choices, specifically about whether and which public employee interests to support. Such mixed or divided organizations weaken the overall political clout of public managers, rendering their efforts to promote public service expansion less likely to succeed.

The historical comparisons of deinstitutionalization in the United States, France, Norway, and Sweden provide empirical evidence for these arguments. Where the managers of public psychiatric institutions lacked an independent and unified political voice (as in the United States and Sweden), their organizations did not form a coalition with the public sector trade unions representing the employees of those institutions. The absence of this political counterweight enabled a series of cutbacks to mental health care that closed hospitals and left few alternatives in their stead. Over time, these cuts also weakened the political power of the public mental health workforce. The opposite occurred in France and Norway. In these two cases, independently organized and unified public mental health care managers and workers formed a coalition with workers to raise wages and protect their employment, and thus the services they provided. Deinstitutionalization there took a different tack, expanding both inpatient and outpatient mental health services and, subsequently, the political power of the public psychiatric workforce. Today, the supply of public mental health services for people with chronic and severe mental illnesses is much higher in France and Norway than in the United States and Sweden. In sum, I have introduced public employees as an explanation for the cross-national variation in mental health care provision, as well as theorized when and why they matter.

THEORETICAL IMPLICATIONS FOR WELFARE STATE SCHOLARSHIP

By exploring the political-economic roots of mental health care variation, I also underline the role of the welfare state as employer, an area insufficiently attended to by theoretical literature in this field.

The Expansion of the "Service Arm" of the Welfare State

Classic theories of welfare state formation have focused on explaining social policies that transfer cash benefits to recipients (the "transfer arm" of the welfare state) but less so on the social policies that structure service provision (the "service arm" of the welfare state). Consider Gøsta Esping-Andersen's canonical *The Three Worlds of Welfare Capitalism* (1990). Esping-Andersen emphasizes the varying influence of political elites on the Left, bolstered by the mass political enfranchisement and unionization of workers during and after industrialization. He finds that the degree of "power resources" historically

TABLE 7.1 *Average public social expenditures on welfare transfers and services in the advanced economies, select years*

	Welfare state spending (% GDP)				
	Transfers and subsidies	Social services			
	(e.g., pensions, unemployment insurance, cash assistance)	Education	Health	Long-term care	*Total*
1930s	5.7	3.3	0.5	–	3.8
1980	13.1	5.2	4.7	0.6	10.5
2014/latest	17	5.2	7.0	1.6	13.8

Note: Figures include data from Australia, Austria, Belgium, Canada, Denmark, Finland, France, Germany, Greece, Ireland, Italy, Japan, the Netherlands, Portugal, Singapore, Spain, Sweden, Switzerland, the United Kingdom, and the United States (Schuknecht 2020).

afforded to the industrial working class produced alternative social benefit systems, conceptualized, however, in terms of pensions, health insurance, and unemployment insurance, or in short, the transfer arm. These transfers were no doubt fundamental to the postwar welfare state.

Yet since that industrial period, the service arm of the welfare state has surged (as Esping-Andersen himself noted in his 1999 sequel publication). In fact, expenditures on social services are rapidly approaching expenditures on transfers and subsidies. As Table 7.1 shows, this latter group, comprising policies such as pensions, unemployment insurance, and cash assistance, once accounted for much of welfare spending. That share, though, has diminished as services like education, health, and long-term care have expanded. Note, furthermore, that actual spending on the transfer arm may be even lower in reality. As the analyst Ludger Schuknecht, former Deputy Secretary-General of the OECD and Chief Economist at the German Ministry of Finance, put it: "most transfers and some subsidies serve the achievement of social objectives; other subsidies support, for example, certain industries" (Schuknecht 2020, 47). In other words, even if these data overestimate the size of welfare-specific transfers and subsidies (and underestimate that of services, see below), the average contemporary welfare state still allocates almost half of its support to its service arm.

The expansion of social services since the postwar period aligns with broader trends in the macro-economy. Across the advanced economies since the 1970s, the locus of economic production has shifted from the industrial sector to the service sector, which today accounts for on average two-thirds of their GDP. This transition has meant that ordinary people now are much more likely to find work providing services at a hospital, school, restaurant, shop, or bank than producing goods at a factory. Social services, in particular, have become prominent areas of output. According to Schuknecht (2020), health care and education on average accounted for less than 6 percent of GDP in 1960 (not shown), but that number has doubled to more than 12 percent today. Caregiving services for children, disabled adults, and the elderly have also mushroomed. Since 1980, long-term care alone has risen from 0.6 to 1.6 percent of GDP, with no indication of slowing down. Taken together, these figures for education, health, and long-term care indicate that advanced economies spend about 14 percent of their GDP on social services; and that is a conservative estimate, as it excludes other important services such as childcare.

These averages about the growing size of the social service sector, though, mask wide and non-negligible differences across and within countries. For scholars of comparative social policy, what is perhaps most notable is that these differences do not align with their usual theoretical expectations. Table 7.1 also compares average public expenditures on health, education, and long-term care across the advanced economies. When aggregated together, spending in these three areas in fact exceeds spending on transfers and subsidies in several countries, including those assumed to have smaller welfare states such as Australia, Ireland, and the United States. Meanwhile, some of the larger welfare states, such as France and Finland, continue to top the rankings in the transfers and subsidies category, but not in the social services category. When disaggregated by sector, spending patterns in health, education, and long-term care continue to puzzle. For example, expenditures on social services in Germany – a country otherwise known for its moderate level of redistributive transfers and joint reliance on public and private financing – vary widely by type, ranking in the top third in health care, the bottom third in education, and the middle third in long-term care (country-specific data not shown, see Schuknecht 2020).

Welfare state scholars have certainly noted the expansion of the service arm. Substantial efforts have been made to accurately characterize its scale and scope (Alber 1995; Antonnen and Sipilä 1996; Bertin et al. 2021; Castles 2009; Daly and Lewis 2000; Jensen 2008, 2011; Kautto 2002), virtually all of which suggest that the welfare state, as Obinger and Starke (2015, 473) note, "may be increasingly shaped by two different political logics at once – an old logic of the transfer state and a new politics of the service state." With the exception of Gingrich (2011), however, few attempts have been made to theoretically develop this new logic.

The Expansion of Public Employment

As the service arm of the welfare state has grown, so too has public employment. Modern public services emerged long before contemporary systems of social transfers, and decisions made about their structure and organization in the late 19th and early 20th centuries are still visible today (Ansell and Lindvall 2020). And yet, their quantitative explosion did not occur until the late 20th century. The deindustrialization of the advanced economies, coupled with increasing rates of female labor force participation, motivated governments to both expand service employment and develop alternatives that could compensate for thus far unpaid domestic labor. Expanding public social services helped to achieve these aims, resulting in mass public employment.

Consider the example of early childhood education and schooling. These services can employ nonindustrial workers (especially women and those at high risk of unemployment), as well as relieve parents, especially mothers, from the responsibility of caring for their young children and free them to pursue careers in the formal labor market instead. The services often depend on public funding (e.g., the US Head Start program) and, in many cases, are fully government-owned and operated (e.g., much of the French crèche system). It is because of growth trends in services like these that public employment in the advanced economies has doubled since 1960 from approximately 6 to 12 percent of the working-age population (Brady et al. 2020, author's calculations).

It is therefore no coincidence that public sector workers began to matter for mental health policy around the time of psychiatric deinstitutionalization. Reinforcing the transformation of mental health was a concurrent one in the labor market. As the advanced economies shifted their emphasis from industry to services, so too did the nature of work (Wren 2013). Moreover, the state provided many of these services directly (Cameron 1978; Lindert 2004). Sectors such as education and health ballooned, the legal rights of public servants expanded, and the unionization membership of public servants climbed, in sharp contrast to the patterns of decline in the industrial private sector. These trends have expanded the influence of public sector workers across postindustrial societies.

Pressures have become especially acute in the Nordic countries, where large-scale public employment supports generous social policy commitments (Esping-Andersen 1990; Iversen and Wren 1998). Scholarship on the less generous welfare states has also emphasized the growing political influence of public employees, including in the United States, where it is perhaps most notable (Freeman 1988; Garrett and Way 1999; Lipsky 1980; Moe 2011).

Recent waves of hostility toward public workers make it clear that these workers occupy a critical, but controversial, role in the labor market. Often viewed as the characteristic labor market "insiders" who benefit from stable, protected employment, government employees have become the targets of both outsiders and the political Right (Emmenegger et al. 2012; Rueda 2007). The assaults perhaps have been fiercest, as well as most successful, in the United States (Ahlquist 2012; Cramer 2016; Hochschild 2018) but they are prominent across OECD countries. Notably, the circumstances of the Nordic welfare states have produced political tensions between public and private employees (Iversen and Wren 1998). Consider, too, the protests by those who feel "left behind" by their economies and governments. If not outright resentful, their relationship to public employees is at a minimum uneasy. Such has been the case of, for example, the *Gilets jaunes* in France, where the large public service is not impervious to attacks either.

That public employment has universally expanded does not mean that welfare workers are universally influential. Not all social service employees are government employees, not all are unionized, and not all are well-protected labor market insiders. For example, scholars of the "worlds" of welfare have already observed that some countries are more likely to provide public social services than others. The large Nordic welfare states have used public service employment to ensure a broad tax base and maintain wage equality, a move that led to both greater female labor force participation and less fiscal discipline, while continental European and anglophone welfare states have not made that choice and instead encouraged private (social and other) service employment to develop (Huber and Stephens 2000; Iversen and Wren 1998). These policy decisions have empowered and disempowered welfare workers, respectively. Moreover, public unionization rates vary widely by policy area, country, and even within and across levels of government. Other measures of labor's influence, such as collective bargaining coverage, vary as well. Linking these variations in the political power of social service employees to the supply of social services, then, is a central contribution of this book.

The Political Logic of Social Service Distribution

One factor that makes the political logic of welfare services different from the political logic of welfare transfers, then, is the emergence of a welfare workforce. Although canonical work on the formation of welfare states emphasized the central role of trade unions, it was principally concerned with the effect of private sector trade unions on the distribution of income transfers such as pensions, unemployment insurance, and cash assistance (e.g., Esping-Andersen 1990; Huber and Stephens 2001). Analyses of the evolution and possible retrenchment of the welfare state have tended to focus on these benefits, too (e.g., Pierson 1996). Yet services and their providers are just as important to the welfare state (e.g., Giaimo 2002; Gingrich 2011; Immergut 1992).

Differences in the distribution of services and transfers are central to understanding their differing politics. As demonstrated in the preceding chapters, the demand for and pressures on public services can be different from those of redistributive policies. Although many social services do serve large, powerful constituencies (see Gingrich 2011), often their beneficiaries can be more diffuse, less organized, and, importantly, politically and socially disenfranchised. Non-voting-age children cannot demand more public schooling. Frail elderly adults cannot organize a campaign to expand care homes. People who are geographically disempowered – such as those in rural areas, low-income neighborhoods, and democratically unincorporated territories – are perpetually "underserved."

Such patterns are quite unlike those found in the transfer state, where unionized voters can make their demands for insurance and other labor market protections clear. Moreover, services face several cost-reduction pressures that transfers do not. For example, related or automated services can become formidable competitors. Neither are services able to compete with wage increases in more productive sectors (Baumol and Bowen 1966). Public services, in particular, are subject to political deregulation and cost-containment initiatives. Each of these factors incentivize service providers to reduce costs, especially in their most expensive budget line: labor and wages. Often facing weak demand and severe cost pressures, then, the employees of public social services are sometimes the only actors with a political stake in maintaining them. That welfare workers have a vested interest in the structure and financing of social policy, though, does not guarantee they will get their way. Only under certain conditions do they achieve their aims.

Like the industrial workers central to classic welfare state scholarship, the "power resources" of public service employees also can vary.
The political resources available to public service employees can take
three broad forms. The first is a familiar one to the classic literature:
their partisanship. Although the industrial working class once served as
the bedrock of center left and social democratic parties, the public sector workforce in fact has now largely assumed this role (Benedetto et al.
2020). In some ways, their power as voters is even more consequential
than that of their industrial counterparts. By electing officials who favor
them, public sector union members appoint their future bargaining partners (Moe 2006). In patronage-oriented societies, furthermore, elected
officials can reward loyal groups with generous public sector positions,
pay, and protections. Such patterns can shape the direction and distribution of social services as well (see, e.g., Ascoli 2011; Costabile 2009;
Sotiropoulos, 2004; also Ferrera 1996).

This book, though, emphasizes that public employees also can exert
influence as workers, not just as voters. A second power resource, then,
is whether the institutional context favors welfare workers. Variations in
institutional context can include the presence of unions and labor laws
that facilitate worker organization, the kinds of contracts that regulate
public employment, the ability of managers to access political and policy
levers to secure financing, and the degree of labor mobility between the
public and private sector. These variations can influence the distribution of social services at the national level, local level, and across policy
areas. Research on the eurozone crisis, for example, found that high deficit countries with unilateral systems of public sector wage-setting (where
government authorities determine pay through laws or administrative
acts) applied more intense cuts than those with more conventional bargaining systems, with consequences for social service provision in those
countries (Bach and Bordogna 2013; Molina 2014). Patterns of historical
development have an impact as well. Consider the example of American
mental health policy: The slow and staggered acquisition of collective
bargaining rights across the states delayed the advocacy of public sector
trade unions on behalf of public psychiatry.

A third set of power resources available to welfare workers are their
political allies. In the same way that coalitions matter to the transfer
state, so too do they matter to the service state. As shown here, coalitions
of social service administrators and unionized public service workers
may now anchor the service state in ways similar to how left politicians
and unionized private sector workers once anchored the transfer state.

In so doing, this book builds on the branch of scholarship in comparative political economy that uncovered preference alignments between managers and workers in the private sector (e.g., Gourevitch and Shinn 2007; Mares 2003; Martin and Swank 2012; Swenson 2002; Thelen 2004). In fact, the circumstances of government employment appear to favor these alignments even more so. "In the public sector," Ahlquist (2017, 417) writes, "there is no profit to divide between workers and capital owners." Wage growth and employment security can benefit public workers as much as they do their managers. As a result, workers and managers in the public sector often find political common ground. But this and other intra-provider politics are only the tip of the iceberg. A range of other work-related factors could condition the influence of the welfare workforce. In examining these links, there is an opportunity to more robustly integrate the scholarship on employment relations with the scholarship on the welfare state, an important intellectual project (Di Carlo 2019) to which this book contributes.

COMPLEX IMPLICATIONS FOR PUBLIC POLICY

The core insight of this book is that public employees have the ability to expand public services for vulnerable populations. On its face, this point may seem like a social policy win-win: Protecting public sector jobs also protects public services for the marginalized. But in fact the policy implications of this point are many and complex. Five areas merit special attention.

First, increasing the supply of public services is a necessary, but not sufficient, condition for improving their quality. To improve the quality of a service, governments must first provide that service. High-quality public services, furthermore, require substantial resources, financial and otherwise. Unlike other sectors, where the level of quality is more likely to benefit from cost-saving technological advancements (Iversen and Wren 1998), the service sector requires ample funding to maintain its quality. The daily, interpersonal experiences of clients and staff depend on many other factors as well. Prejudices, for example, are well-documented (e.g., FitzGerland and Hurst 2017; Hall et al. 2015; Pit-ten Cate and Glock 2019). In addition, the economic and psychological demands of service work make it especially vulnerable to time constraints and burnout, neither of which contributes positively to quality outcomes. In short, client satisfaction likely increases if staff benefit from secure, well-paid work; but it does not guarantee it.

Second, increasing the supply of public services may or may not be morally desirable. This study focuses on the expansion of the welfare state, which some may already view with a skeptical eye (Piven and Cloward 1979). But in addition, some forms of public employment can contribute to the expansion of the punitive state. The same coalitions that I observe in the mental health sector could also shape the carceral system, the police force, and the military. Note also how, within each of the countries in this study, the scale of public service provision varies across policy areas, with alternative consequences for mental health itself. Although both the United States and Sweden reduced the supply of mental health care, different services "compensate" for this absence: prisons in the United States, social care in Sweden. These differences can produce opposite experiences for people living with psychiatric conditions in each country.

Third, the impact of public employment on socioeconomic inequality is mixed. Governments can use this sector to achieve several social aims, including full employment, job security, and macroeconomic wage equality (Iversen and Wren 1998). Moreover, in comparison to the private sector, the public sector disproportionately employs those who are often excluded from the labor market. These groups include women, racial and ethnic minorities, and people with disabilities (European Commission 2010; Laird 2017; Wilson et al. 2015). They can also expect their pay to be closer to that of their male, non-minoritized, and non-disabled counterparts in the public sector than elsewhere, in part because government employers are more likely to rely on a standardized wage scale than private employers.

In some ways, however, the expansion of public sector work has aggravated these inequalities. The rise of "dualization" in many economies has split labor market participants into two camps: the insiders, who benefit from standard employment, and the outsiders, who do not. For the insiders, work is full-time, continuous, long-term, as well as remunerated above levels of subsistence (Mückenberger 1985 in Seeleib-Kaiser et al. 2012). This form of employment, though once the model of postwar male industrial work, is now perhaps best maintained in public services. Meanwhile, labor market outsiders are especially vulnerable to unemployment and subject to jobs with poor pay, protections, and employment rights (Rueda 2014). Although these divides partly explain the political divide between the "left behind" and public employees, it is important to emphasize that women, young people, and (often racialized) low-skilled workers tend to be overrepresented as outsiders as well (Häusermann and Schwander 2012).[2] In this

---

[2] For work that inverts the assumption that the populist challenge stems from outsiders (but rather from threatened insiders), see Häusermann (2020).

way, public employment is a manifestation, not a solution, of the structural inequalities that pervade contemporary labor markets.

Fourth, this rift in the welfare state's support base could have far-reaching implications. A political competition is brewing. On the Left, public and other service employees advocate for the services that either directly employ them or support the caregiving services that they cannot provide for their own households; but their sheltered positions in the labor market allow them to either take the traditional forms of social protection for granted or otherwise opt out of solidaristic insurance schemes that pool risks with workers in other sectors (Rehm 2020).[3] The industrial working class, on the Right, may favor traditional social protection but it also eschews the expansion of public social services, often driven by ethnocentric and gendered resentment. This contestation may produce a trade-off for welfare states. Countries with politically powerful public employees, for example, may develop universalistic public services at the expense of redistributive cash benefits. In any event, whether and how politicians respond to this competition with concrete policy change is an ongoing and highly salient question for contemporary welfare states.

This shift has significant implications for the political basis of – and hence demands on – the welfare state. The newer left party voters tend to privilege "social investment" policies such as childcare and education over the traditional compensatory policies such as unemployment insurance (Gingrich and Häusermann 2015). Social democrats, in an attempt to reformulate party positions, have responded by alienating their former base (Mudge 2018; Oesch and Rennwald 2018). As the traditional working class gravitates toward radical right parties, meanwhile, so too do the positions of their politicians on particular aspects of social policy. Many of these parties have adopted a "welfare chauvinist" attitude that favors the white, male breadwinner model of social policy (Betz 1994; Mudde 2000; Rathgeb 2021).

Fifth, scholars should pay attention to whether and how public employment shapes macroeconomic performance and, by extension,

---

[3] That women's formal employment in public social services has replaced their informal care of the needy (such as the mentally ill) reveals the endogenous relationship between the revolution of women's roles and welfare state development. As women leave the home and enter the labor market, demands for family caregiving increase. These demands prompt the expansion of a formal labor market to provide these public services. Because this new labor market tends to employ women, it diminishes informal family caregiving capacity further and continues to spur demand for public provision of this care. Thanks go to Gøsta Esping-Andersen for this point, raised in personal correspondence in September 2022.

the financial underpinnings of the welfare state itself. Reservations about fiscal discipline are warranted (Iversen and Wren 1998), but the precise effect of high public spending on economic performance often depends on other factors, such as the proportion of dependents (van der Ploeg 2007) or the structure and capacities of the tax system (Andersen and Kreiner 2017). Moreover, increasing public spending can reduce levels of inequality and promote economic growth (Cingano 2014; Pontusson and Baccaro 2020). Complicating this picture is the fact that many governments have supplemented conventional public financing tools (e.g., fiscal policy) with contemporary alternatives (e.g., public and private debt). This trend reflects the demands of tax-conscious voters, as well as the prerogatives of neoliberal, banking-centric capitalism. This shift has contributed to a much more profound political-economic crisis that lacks easy solutions (Streeck 2013, 2017). Understanding the long-term implications of expanded public employment, then, requires giving careful, context-specific attention to these macroeconomic complexities.

TOWARD GOOD JOBS AND GOOD SERVICES

The face of social policy is changing, with profound implications for its recipients. Increased expenditures on social services, such as health clinics or schools, may shape an individual's experience of the welfare state more intimately than a deposited pension or unemployment check. Social service provision can involve complex, repeated, and extended interactions with a myriad of providers. These providers, as shown, play an important role forming the public policies that structure those services. How this phenomenon – the political logic of social service provision – shapes the lives of the most vulnerable populations cannot be ignored.

Robust public services require robust public unions. They require government funds and protections for the workers providing those services. Otherwise, public services are unsustainable. Neither policy analysts nor client advocates should dismiss the demands of workers to protect services as simply efforts to retain their employment. We instead should be mindful of services' dual role. Like the picket signs hoisted in Billiers (see Chapter 1) asserted, public services support both "jobs" and "health" (or human well-being more generally). To that end, policy proposals that conflate reform with abolition, such as the most extreme versions of deinstitutionalization, should be reviewed with caution. Retrenchment can sometimes balance budgets but rarely does it redress social needs.

To optimize the symbiotic relationship between public services and public unions, a cooperative approach is vital. Both workers and clients need a seat at the decision-making table. In this book, Norway's Council for Mental Health embodied this principle best. An organization that represented all the relevant groups of welfare workers and collaborated with managers, it also included client advocates in its deliberations. The Council's efforts paid off impressively in the mental health care reforms that followed. Today, Norway's comprehensive mental health care system is known for both its full suite of psychiatric medical services (ranging from outpatient to inpatient) and its innovative programs inspired by user experiences, such as its drug-free treatment centers.

Collaboration across policy sectors is also important. Developing flexible education and training systems, for example, can help welfare workers in health care adapt to evolving client needs, demographic changes, and technological developments. In fact, this cross-sectoral approach is a model for social policy systems as a whole. The design of most welfare states reflects the priorities and worlds of their founders, who created them decades ago. Few have adjusted to the social trends that have emerged since then. Like population mental health, which encompasses an increasingly broad range of conditions, other issues – such as climate concerns, new family structures, and migration – improve most when multiple policy areas work in tandem to address them. Here, too, alliances are key.

Postscript

The Evolving Definition of the "Welfare Workforce"

Scholars and policy-makers interested in exploring and applying the insights of this book to current events should be mindful of the evolving definition of the "welfare workforce." Throughout this book, I have defined public sector workers as those who are directly employed by national or local governments and depend on government funds for most of their wages. That definition is suitable for the policy area and time period of interest.

A highly polarized medical specialty, mental health care faces a sharp public/private divide. Its clients are either unable to afford costly long-term treatments (and thus rely on public generosity) or sufficiently moneyed to cover the substantial out-of-pocket health and social care costs associated with mental illness. Psychiatric workers tend to serve one clientele or the other, thereby depending on government funds for their wages either heavily or hardly at all. Moreover, the distinction between public and private mental health workers was especially clear during the period of psychiatric deinstitutionalization; the large-scale delegation of social welfare services to private and not-for-profit actors was not yet underway. This trend, though now a common feature of mature welfare states, developed only in the late 20th and early 21st centuries. By then, the mental health transformation had begun, with a discernible role for government employees.

The boundaries between public and private welfare are becoming ever less clear, especially in policy areas where clients are less vulnerable. Over the past several decades, governments have introduced a variety of market-based mechanisms into public services (Gingrich 2011), delegated social protection to private actors (Hackett 2020; Mettler

2011; Morgan and Campbell 2011; Mori 2020), and financialized provision through private instruments (Naczyk 2013; Thurston 2018; van der Zwan 2014). In fact, just as welfare services have become more comprehensive, so too has their reliance on decentralized authority and privatization (Bode 2017). Moreover, the distinction between income transfers and in-kind services is blurring; beneficiaries often use pensions, tax credits, and vouchers for health, education, and childcare services (Martinelli 2017). The result is an entangled web of overlapping public and private jurisdictions that complicates the identities of welfare workers.

In fact, labor market dualization is occurring not just between the welfare workforce and other occupational groups but also within the welfare workforce itself (Hermann and Flecker 2015; Mori 2020). Protected, stable public sector employment benefits some welfare workers, in particular high-skilled professionals in interpersonal professions, such as health and education (see Oesch 2006). At the same time, newer, and frequently outsourced, services often lack these protections. The care sector is a case in point (Martinelli et al. 2017). The increasing demand for child and elderly care has expanded non-state provision of these services, which are often provided by low-skilled, immigrant women (especially where labor market regulations, wages, and unionization rates are lower, see Morgan 2005). Although public subsidies may support these services, the employees delivering them do not always benefit from the same protections and pay available to other welfare workers.

Consider for example how contemporary bargaining regimes governing nonprofit or contracted social service work may influence policy in ways different from those governing public sector work (e.g., Finger and Lastra-Anadón 2021; Salamon 1995). Subsequent scholarship might examine how these different bargaining regimes shape the content of social services, as well as how effects may differ by level of government or by policy area.[1] What is more, the scope of bargaining or the availability of alternative levers could allow workers to influence policy in ways

---

[1] Note also that the typologies of public sector wage bargaining may or may not be linked to existing patterns of labor and economic relations. For instance, one proposed typology finds that the "varieties" of public sector wage bargaining do not align with the distinction between liberal and coordinated market economies proposed by the Varieties of Capitalism literature (Bach and Bordogna 2019). More research is needed to examine why, as well as to see whether and how these patterns apply to typologies of social service provision (see, e.g., Jensen 2008; Stoy 2014).

that go beyond pay and into other areas, such as gender equity and safe staffing (Bach and Bordogna 2019).

Updated definitions of public sector work, then, should consider a variety of context-specific questions. For example, are the relevant employees subject to public or private labor law? To that end, is the legal status of charitable, not-for-profit, or third sector providers distinct? How do welfare workers interact with other labor market institutions, such as vocational training or collective bargaining? Are the relevant licensing and entrance procedures unique to the public service, or are they transferable to the private sector? Furthermore, to what extent is the role of the state visible to these workers? Indeed, social policy may be "hidden" from welfare workers in the same way that it can be "hidden" from recipients (see Howard 1997; Mettler 2005; Morgan and Campbell 2011). How governments license, finance, and contract social services, then, could shape how scholars classify their employees.

Appendix

Comparative Deinstitutionalization Data Set – Codebook and Source Information

DESCRIPTION AND AIMS

This original database compares the process of psychiatric deinstitution-alization across 16 advanced economies with standardized, cross-national data from 1935 to at least 1990. As such, the data allows researchers to better understand the varying patterns of change in mental health care services over time as well as across countries.

As noted in Chapter 2, these countries are the first movers: societies whose early industrialization prompted the rise of the asylum, and whose extraordinary economic prosperity in the 20th century prompted its decline. Their national trends eventually set the international standard. To quantitatively delineate the universe of cases, I selected the most affluent democracies of the postwar period by examining their GDP per capita in 1960. According to the Comparative Welfare States Data Set (Brady et al. 2020), this indicator exceeded $12,000 in all countries, averaging around $17,000 in the set (standard deviation: about $4,000, all amounts standardized to contemporary USD; per BLS 2023). A relatively tight distribution, the next wealthiest country on the list (Italy) is almost a full standard deviation (0.7) less than the lowest unit in the range (Finland). Italy is nonetheless included because its 1978 Basaglia law gained attention as a bellwether of the international deinstitutional-ization movement (Donnelly 1992; Foot 2015). Moreover, the law was a byproduct of earlier deinstitutionalization trends in the more indus-trialized North, which paralleled those of the other countries in this study. Italy's spatially unequitable economic development likely delayed the law's adoption at the national level. Countries with a population less than 1 million (micro-states) are excluded from the dataset (e.g., Luxembourg).

The dates of the data set span the full-time period during which mental health services transformed. The Second World War was a major turning point in the history of social welfare: The spirit of reform, combined with an economic boom, made for considerable policy changes, especially in the area of mental health. The development of social insurance funds, the increasing medicalization of psychiatry, and the return of war veterans facing profound psychological distress prompted reforms in the asylum. Because this flurry of activity occurred after the war, the series begins in 1935 to obtain a baseline measure of institutionalization. Tracking the series through 1990 captures the effects of the welfare retrenchment since the economic crises of the 1970s, which also prompted reductions in psychiatric care supply. Data on psychiatric hospitals and residents, for example, were much more prevalent in the earlier period than in the later period, when countries started to replace those numbers with data on psychiatric beds and inpatients.

To obtain the requisite information, a research team surveyed national statistical yearbooks for the full universe of cases from 1935 to 1990, supplemented by other official government reports as well as data from the WHO and OECD. Data was recorded in approximately five-year increments, or as otherwise noted. The series mostly describes changes in public (not private) institutions. Country-by-country details about context-specific definitions, measurement, data collection patterns, and source information are provided in the following table.

Country	Residents	Mental hospitals	Psychiatric beds	Comments	Source(s)
Australia	1935–41: Number of patients on books at end of year in hospitals for the insane 1945–60: Number of patients on books at end of year in mental hospitals 1965: Mental patients on the register at June 30 1970–75 Number of inpatients at end of year in mental health institutions 2005: Estimated number of residents in residential mental health care	1935–41: Number of hospitals for the insane 1945–60: Number of mental hospitals 1965–74: Psychiatric centers, psychiatric hospitals, and mental hospitals (excludes institutions labeled "private," in particular the New South Wales private psychiatric centers) 1990–2012: (Number of) public psychiatric hospitals	1935–41: Number of beds and cots in hospitals for the insane 1945–60: Number of beds and cots in mental hospitals 1965–70: Number of beds and cots for patients in mental health inpatient institutions 1990–2000: Available beds in public psychiatric hospitals 2005: Mental health hospital beds in public psychiatric hospitals 2012: Beds in public psychiatric hospitals	Since most of the earlier data (1935–60) appear to exclude data on private institutions, we continued to exclude private institutions for subsequent years (1965–2012). Data for private institutions, though, is available for most of those more recent years as well.	Commonwealth Bureau of Census and Statistics, *Official Yearbook of the Commonwealth of Australia* (1935–2012).

(continued)

207

Country	Residents	Mental hospitals	Psychiatric beds	Comments	Source(s)
Austria	Series unavailable	1937: We manually counted all mental hospitals (public and private) in the source book 1951–66: Institutions for nervous and mental illnesses (observations include those both with and without public rights) 1976–90: Institutions for nervous and mental illnesses	1937: We manually counted all beds in the mental hospitals (public and private) identified in the source book 1951–66: Beds in institutions for nervous and mental illnesses (observations include those both with and without public rights) 1976–90: Beds in institutions for nervous and mental illnesses	Since most of the more recent data (1976–90) appear to include data on private institutions, we also included data on private institutions for previous years (1937–66). Data on public institutions only is nonetheless available for most of those earlier years as well.	Ilberg, G., and H. Laehr (Eds.). 1937. *Die Anstalten für Geisteskranke, Nervenkranke, Schwachsinnige, Epileptische, Trunksüchtige usw. In Deutschland, Österreich und der Schweiz einschließlich der psychiatrischen und neurologischen wissenschaftlichen Institute.* Berlin and Leipzig: Walter de Gruyter & Co. Österreichischen Staatsdruckerei, Statistisches Handbuch für die Republik Österreich (1950–90).

Country					Source
Belgium	1935–60: Sick patients establishments for the mentally ill (closed services including the establishments of Geel and Lierneux) 1965–83: Patients in psychiatric establishments (closed service)	Series incomplete (missing 1935–60)	Series incomplete (missing 1935–60)		Institut national de statistique, Ministère des affaires économiques, *Annuaire statistique de la Belgique* (1935–95).
Canada	1935–55: (Total resident) patients in mental institutions (in Canada) at December 31 1959: Patients in public mental hospitals at December 31 1970–82: Average daily number of patients in public mental hospitals	1935–45: All mental institutions except for private mental institutions (includes public hospitals, training schools, psychiatric hospitals, community and municipal institutions, and dominion hospitals classified as "mental institutions")	1935–45: Normal bed capacity in mental institutions in Canada 1950–75: Beds in public mental institutions 1978: Beds in (reporting) public mental hospitals on January 1	Although data on private institutions is often available, we privileged the (more commonly) available data on public institutions.	Dominion Bureau of Statistics, *The Canada Year Book* (1935–90).

(continued)

(continued)

Country	Residents	Mental hospitals	Psychiatric beds	Comments	Source(s)
		1950: Public mental institutions 1955–75: Public mental hospitals 1978: (Reporting) public mental hospitals 1986: Number of mental hospitals (excludes Prince Edward Island, Yukon, and NW Territories; data for Quebec includes allied special, rehabilitation, and extended care hospitals)			
Denmark	Complete series not available	1935: State mental hospitals 1945–75: State, municipal, and private mental (psychiatric) hospitals	1945–75: Beds in state, municipal, and private mental (psychiatric) hospitals 1985–95: Beds in psychiatric hospitals, total		Danmarks Statistik, *Statistisk Årbog.* (1937–97).

(continued)

| Finland | 1935–55: Male and female mental defectives in state hospitals, private hospitals, communal hospitals, private hospitals, communal institutions, and private homes 1988: Since resident data is not available for the end of the series, we estimate it for this year. Average length of stay remained high in Finland (125.1 days this year), so we interpret the bed occupancy rate multiplied by the number of mental hospital beds as an acceptable, if imperfect, indicator of the resident population in this year | 1936–40: Total number of state, municipal, and private mental hospitals in cities and in the countryside 1945–90: Total number of state, communal, and private mental hospitals | 1935: Since bed data is not available for the beginning of the series, we estimate it for this year. In the years following the Second World War (1945–50), beds in mental hospitals accounted for about 30 percent (29.6–30.02 percent) of the total number of beds in Finland. The psychiatric bed estimate for 1935 is 30 percent of the total number of general and other hospital beds in that year. 1945–90: Number of beds in state, communal, and private mental hospitals | Although data is often subdivided by institutional type (e.g., state, communal, or private hospital; as well as charity and in-home care), it is not consistently so. We hence provide data for all psychiatric institutions, though most services are provided at the municipal (communal) level. Note also that the population residing in psychiatric care often doubles the number of psychiatric beds. The reason for this discrepancy is unclear; however, it appears that during this period some residential care was available in non-hospital institutions (e.g., charities and private homes). | Tilastokeskus, *Suomen tilastollinen vuosikirja* (1935–2000). |

211

Country	Residents	Mental hospitals	Psychiatric beds	Comments	Source(s)
France	1935–75: Number of patients hospitalized in psychiatric establishments on December 31 of each year 1985–88: Patients (*malades*) present on January 1 (in psychiatric establishments)	1933: National and departmental asylums, hospices, and private asylums 1955: Psychiatric hospitals 1964–96: Public psychiatric hospitals (or specialized psychiatric hospital center) and private psychiatric hospitals acting as public institutions	1935: We infer this observation from Lauzier and Lafage (1958, 439), who note that 1,740 psychiatric beds had been added since the interwar period. We hence subtract that number from the 1955 observation to estimate the number of psychiatric beds in this year 1955: Number of beds in psychiatric hospitals 1970–75: Number of beds in public psychiatric hospitals (or specialized psychiatric hospital centers), psychiatric wards in public hospitals, private sanatoriums (*maisons de santé*), and private psychiatric hospitals acting as public institutions		Institut national de la statistique et des études économiques. *Annuaire statistique de la France* (1935–2007). Lauzier and Lafage (1958) Meslé and Vallin (1981)

Germany					
1935: Inpatients (*Krankenbestand*) on December 31 in hospitals for the mentally ill and epileptics 1995: Cases in psychiatric facilities (preventive and rehabilitative care), excludes neurology, psychosomatic, and addiction care	1935: Sanatoriums and nursing homes for the mentally ill, epileptics, etc., including those who also suffer from nervous disorders, etc. 1995: Total number of hospitals specializing in psychiatry or psychiatry and neurological beds	1985–96: Number of beds in public psychiatric hospitals (or specialized psychiatric hospital centers), private sanatoriums (*maisons de santé*), and private psychiatric hospitals acting as public institutions	1935: Number of regular hospital beds at the end of the year for hospitals for the mentally ill and epileptics 1995: Beds in total number of hospitals specializing in psychiatry or psychiatry and neurological beds	Although the source reports data on the Federal Republic of Germany (West Germany) during the postwar period, it excludes information on the German Democratic Republic (East Germany) during this time. For this reason, we include only data from periods of unification (before and after the split).	*Statistischen Reichsamt/ Statistischen Bundesamtes, Statistisches Jahrbuch für Das Deutsche Reich/ Statistisches Jahrbuch für die Bundesrepublik Deutschland (1935→95).*

(continued)

(*continued*)

Country	Residents	Mental hospitals	Psychiatric beds	Comments	Source(s)
Great Britain	1938: Registered persons of unsound mind at January 1 in Institutions provided by County and Borough Councils under the Lunacy Acts in England, Wales, and Scotland (excludes state criminal lunatic asylums and other institutions under the Poor Laws, since their purposes went beyond the medical and custodial to include punishment, commodification, etc.; also excludes data on Northern Ireland for better comparability with the latter part of the series)	Complete series unavailable	Complete series unavailable	See Jones (1983) on the challenges of collecting historical data on mental health services in the United Kingdom of Great Britain and Northern Ireland. In brief, the Mental Health Act of 1959 significantly altered the basis on which mental health statistics were gathered, rendering the statistical figures before and after that year difficult to compare. Moreover, tables on key variables are often aggregated and disaggregated in succeeding years. For example, sometimes Wales and England are presented together, other times not; "psychiatric services" may or may not include services for the mentally handicapped, and children and people over the age of 65 are sometimes included or excluded;	Central Statistical Office, *Annual Abstract of Statistics* (1938–90). Government Statistical Service. *Health and Personal Social Services Statistics for England* (1978). Jones (1983).

214

Country			Source	Notes
	1955: Inpatient average daily occupation of beds (mental and mentally deficient) in England, Wales, and Scotland 1960–85: Average daily occupation of beds in psychiatric departments in England and Wales; mental and mentally deficient in Scotland			some localities mix the data on the mentally ill with data those with physical disabilities, mental disabilities, or even lucid but frail elderly. Additional data collection challenges arose after the late 1970s, when budgetary challenges stalled surveillance efforts. The last detailed Mental Health Inquiry for England and Wales was published in 1978 and only includes data up to then. Any other related publications either ceased publishing around this time as well, only base their information on the 1976 data, or give no mental health statistics at all.
Italy	1938–50: Mentally ill patients hospitalized in institutes of assistance on January 1	1955–74: Public neuropsychiatric hospitals 1980–90: Public psychiatric hospitals	1955–74: Beds in public neuropsychiatric hospitals 1980–90: Beds in public psychiatric hospitals	Ministero dell'interno, Direzione generale di statistica, *Annuario statistico italiano* (1935–2000).	Although data on private institutions is available for more recent years, we focused our data collection on public institutions, which has been more consistently available since the 1930s.

(continued)

(continued)

Country	Residents	Mental hospitals	Psychiatric beds	Comments	Source(s)
	1957–74: Patients present at the beginning of the year in public neuropsychiatric hospitals 1980–90: Patients present at the beginning of the year in public psychiatric hospitals				
Netherlands	1935–40: Total (population) on December 31 in institutions for the insane 1945: Total (population) under care (in institutions for the insane)	1935–40: Number of institutions for the insane 1945: Number of mental hospitals 1953–64: Hospitals for mental defectives 1966–88: (Number of) mental hospitals	Complete series unavailable		Centraal Bureau Voor de Statistiek, *Jaarcijfers voor Nederland* (1940–90).

New Zealand	1950–60: (Population) Under care on December 31 in hospitals for mental defectives 1965–70: Patients in mental hospitals on December 31 1970–87: Inpatients in mental hospitals on December 31 1935–50: Number of patients remaining at the end of the year in public mental hospitals and the (one) private mental hospital 1955: Number of patients resident and voluntary boarders in public mental hospitals and the private mental hospital at the end of the year	1935–55: Public mental hospitals and the (one) private mental hospital 1960–65: Mental hospitals (excludes hospitals and training schools for the mentally subnormal) 1990: Psychiatric hospitals	Complete series unavailable	Department of Statistics, *New Zealand Official Yearbook* (1935–90).

(continued)

217

Country	Residents	Mental hospitals	Psychiatric beds	Comments	Source(s)
	1960–65: Average number of resident patients and voluntary boarders on the register (in mental hospitals) 1974–80: Average number of people resident in psychiatric hospitals during year 1985–90: Average number of resident patients in psychiatric hospitals and hospitals for the mentally handicapped				
Norway	1935: Mental health patients treated at asylums (remaining at end of year) 1945: Mental health patients at mental health hospitals at the end of the year	1935: Mental asylums 1945–55: Mental hospitals 1965–85: Psychiatric hospitals (excludes psychiatric nursing homes)	1935: Beds in mental asylums 1945–55: Beds in mental hospitals 1965–85: Beds in psychiatric hospitals (excludes psychiatric nursing homes)	As Chapter 6 discusses, in the postwar period Norway expanded custodial care for elderly psychiatric patients by constructing psychiatric nursing homes. For cross-national consistency (and since these nursing homes served a primarily custodial,	Statistisk sentralbyrå, *Statistisk årbok for Norge* (1937–97).

				Notes	Source
	1965–75: Patients in psychiatric hospitals (in total) at the end of the year 1985: Patient population in psychiatric hospitals, clinic, sanatoria (including the state clinic for drug addicts) at the end of the year		1995: Beds in psychiatric hospitals (including psychiatric departments in somatic hospitals and psychiatric clinics; excludes beds in psychiatric nursing homes)	not medical, function), we excluded data on those institutions, beds, and residents.	
Sweden	Complete series not available	1935–45: Civilian health care facilities – state mental hospitals 1965: State mental hospitals for mentally diseased 1975: Mental hospitals	1935–45: Civilian health care facilities – state mental hospitals: beds 1965: State mental hospitals for mentally diseased: beds 1975: Mental hospitals: beds	Although Sweden developed other forms of institutional care in the postwar period, this series presents data on state mental hospitals, which was consistently collected during the period of interest and provided the largest portion of mental health care during that time.	SCB-Statistiska centralbyrän. *Statistisk årsbok för Sverige* (1937–97).
Switzerland	1936–65: Patients treated in specialized establishments for mental and nervous illness	1936–56: Specialized establishments for patients with mental and nervous illness	1936–65: Beds in specialized establishments for mental and nervous illness		Office fédéral de la statistique. *Annuaire statistique de la Suisse* (1935–98).

(continued)

(*continued*)

Country	Residents	Mental hospitals	Psychiatric beds	Comments	Source(s)
	1983: Hospitalized patients in psychiatric clinics	1965–75: Institutions/ establishments for mental illness 1983: University psychiatric clinics and other psychiatric clinics	1975: Number of beds for the sick in establishments for the mentally ill 1983: Beds in university psychiatric clinics and other psychiatric clinics 1995: Beds in psychiatric clinics		
United States	1935: Patients present on January 1 in state hospitals for mental disease 1950–85: Resident patients at end of year in state and county mental (care) hospitals	1938: State, county, and city hospitals 1950–2000: State and county mental hospitals	Complete series not available	For consistency, our data collection focuses on the population in and absolute number of state and county mental hospitals, the historical anchor of the US mental health system. Some data is periodically available on other public institutions (e.g., federal institutions, veterans; facilities) and private hospitals as well.	National Institute of Mental Health. *Patients in mental institutions* (1938). US Department of Commerce, *Statistical Abstract of the United States* (1935–2000).

President's
Commission on
Mental Health.
*Task Panel
Reports, Volume 2*
(1978).
US Department
of Health and
Human Services,
Substance Abuse
and Mental
Health Services
Administration.
*Mental Health,
United States*
(2002).

Bibliography

UNPUBLISHED SOURCES

Archives

Please see the chapters for citations to the box/folder level.

Archives Nationales (AN). Commission des maladies mentales, 19950173/1; 19910084/28-30. Pierrefitte-sur-Seine.

Riksarkivet. Psykiatriutredningen Korrespondens, SE/RA/324277/E. Stockholm (Marieberg).

Walter P. Reuther Library Archives of Labor and Urban Affairs (RL). AFSCME Publications, LR002503; AFSCME Office of the President: Zander Records, LR001986; AFSCME Office of the President: Wurf Records (WR), LR001987; AFSCME Communications Department Records: Wurf Speeches (WS), LR002204; AFSCME Public Policy and Analysis Department Records (PPAD), main collection on deinstitutionalization, LR002203, LR0001994, and finding aid. Wayne State University, Detroit.

Interviews

Former French civil servant (senior official at the Ministry of Health), March 2018.
Former Swedish civil servant (coauthor of *SOU* 1992:73), August 2022.
Former President of the Swedish Psychiatric Association, June 2022.
Former President of the Norwegian Psychiatric Association, June 2022.
Former Norwegian civil servant (Assistant Director of the Board of Health), July 2022.
Former Norwegian civil servant (Deputy Minister of Health), July 2022.
Former Norwegian civil servant (mental health financing expert), August 2022.
Former Norwegian civil servant (lead author of *NOU* 1995:14), July 2022.
Former Chair of the Norwegian Council for Mental Health, August 2022.
Former Secretary General of the Norwegian Council for Mental Health, August 2022.

PUBLISHED SOURCES

Includes only those abbreviated in-text. Please see the chapters' footnotes for legislative and administrative documents, most newspaper articles and other media, as well as material from trade and professional press.

Ahlquist, John S. 2012. "Public Sector Unions Need the Private Sector or Why the Wisconsin Protests Were Not Labor's Lazarus Moment." *The Forum* 10 (1): 1–17.

Ahlquist, John S. 2017. "Labor Unions, Political Representation, and Economic Inequality." *Annual Review of Political Science* 20 (1): 409–32.

Ahlquist, John S., and Margaret Levi. 2013. *In the Interest of Others: Organizations and Social Activism*. Princeton: Princeton University Press.

Alber, Jens. 1995. "A Framework for the Comparative Study of Social Services." *Journal of European Social Policy* 5 (2): 131–49.

Alesina, Alberto, Arnaud Devleeschauwer, William Easterly, Sergio Kurlat, and Romain Wacziarg. 2003. "Fractionalization." *Journal of Economic Growth* 8 (2): 155–94.

Alfandari, François. 2017. "Le syndicalisme à l'heure de la transformation de la psychiatrie: Des militants CGT à l'hôpital psychiatrique du Vinatier (Lyon, années 1960–1970)." *Genèses* 2 (107): 82–105.

Alfandari, François. 2018. "Produire un syndicalisme 'politique.' La CGT dans un hôpital psychiatrique de 1968 à nos jours." Université Lumière Lyon 2-Université de Lyon.

Allen, Jessica, Reuben Balfour, Ruth Bell, and Michael Marmot. 2014. "Social Determinants of Mental Health." *International Review of Psychiatry* 26 (4): 392–407.

Andersen, Søren Kaj, Christian Lyhne Ibsen, Kristin Alsos, Kristine Nergaard, and Pekka Sauramo. 2015. "Changes in Wage Policy and Collective Bargaining in the Nordic Countries – Comparison of Denmark, Finland, Norway and Sweden." *Wage Bargaining under the New European Economic Governance: Alternative Strategies for Inclusive Growth*, edited by Guy van Gyes and Thorsten Schulten, 139–68. Brussels: European Trade Union Institute.

Andersen, Torben M., and Claus T. Kreiner. 2017. "Baumol's Cost Disease and the Sustainability of the Welfare State." *Economica* 84 (335): 417–29.

Anderson, Karen M., and Julia Lynch. 2007. "Reconsidering Seniority Bias: Aging, Internal Institutions, and Union Support for Pension Reform." *Comparative Politics* 39 (2): 189–208.

Anell, Anders, Anna H. Glenngård, and Sherry Merkur. 2012. "Sweden: Health System Review." *Health Systems in Transition* 14 (5), 1–159.

Ansell, Ben W., and Johannes Lindvall. 2020. *Inward Conquest: The Political Origins of Modern Public Services*. Cambridge Studies in Comparative Politics. Cambridge: Cambridge University Press.

Anttonen, Anneli, and Jorma Sipilä. 1996. "European Social Care Services: Is It Possible To Identify Models?" *Journal of European Social Policy* 6 (2): 87–100.

Anzia, Sarah F., and Terry M. Moe. 2016. "Do Politicians Use Policy to Make Politics? The Case of Public-Sector Labor Laws." *American Political Science Review* 110 (4): 763–77.

Arthur, Brian. 1994. *Increasing Returns and Path Dependence in the Economy*. Ann Arbor: University of Michigan Press.

Ascoli, Ugo, editor. 2011. *Il Welfare in Italia*. Bologna: Il Mulino.

Atay, Joanne E., Raquel Crider, Daniel Foley, Alisa A. Male, and Beatrice Blacklow. 2006. "Background Report, Admissions and Resident Patients, State and County Mental Hospitals, United States, 2004." US Department of Health and Human Services, Substance Abuse and Mental Health Services Administration, Center for Mental Health Services.

Auerbach, Adam Michael. 2019. *Demanding Development: The Politics of Public Goods Provision in India's Urban Slums*. Cambridge Studies in Comparative Politics. Cambridge: Cambridge University Press.

Ayme, Jean. 1995. *Chroniques de la psychiatrie publique: à travers l'histoire d'un syndicat*. Collection "Des Travaux et des Jours." Ramonville-Saint-Agne: Editions Érès.

Baccaro, Lucio, and Chris Howell. 2017. *Trajectories of Neoliberal Transformation: European Industrial Relations since the 1970s*. Cambridge: Cambridge University Press.

Bach, Stephen, and Lorenzo Bordogna. 2013. "Reframing Public Service Employment Relations: The Impact of Economic Crisis and the New EU Economic Governance." *European Journal of Industrial Relations* 19 (4): 279–94.

Bach, Stephen, and Lorenzo Bordogna. 2019. "Public Employers: What Is Distinctive about Public Sector Wage Setting and Why Does It Matter?" For the Max Planck Institute for the Study of Societies "Political Economy of Public Sector Wage Setting" Conference, Cologne.

Bachrach, Leona L. 1983. "An Overview of Deinstitutionalization." *New Directions for Mental Health Services* 1983 (17): 5–14.

Baldwin, Peter. 1992. *The Politics of Social Solidarity: Class Bases of the European Welfare State, 1875–1975*. Cambridge: Cambridge University Press.

Bambra, Clare. 2005. "Worlds of Welfare and the Health Care Discrepancy." *Social Policy and Society* 4 (1): 31–41.

Barnard, Alexander. 2019a. "Bureaucratically Split Personalities: (Re)ordering the Mentally Disordered in the French State." *Theory and Society* 48: 753–84.

Barnard, Alexander. 2019b. "Ordering the Disordered: State Classifications of Mental Illness in France and the United States." Doctoral thesis, University of California, Berkeley.

Barton, Walter E. 1987. *The History and Influence of the American Psychiatric Association*. Washington, DC: American Psychiatric Press.

Bauduret, Jean-François. 2002. "Chronique sur 35 ans de sectorisation psychiatrique: 1960–1995." *Rhizome* 9 (September): 3–4.

Bauduret, Jean-François. 2022. "Plus de 60 ans de sectorisation psychiatrie: de l'esprit des textes à la réalité des pratiques." *Pratiques en santé mentale* 68 (4): 11–7.

Baumol, William J., and William G. Bowen. 1966. *Performing Arts – The Economic Dilemma: A Study of Problems Common to Theater, Opera, Music and Dance*. New York: The Twentieth Century Fund.

Bayer, Ronald. 1987. *Homosexuality and American Psychiatry: The Politics of Diagnosis*. Princeton Paperbacks. Princeton: Princeton University Press.

Béland, Daniel, and Edella Schlager. 2019. "Varieties of Policy Feedback Research: Looking Backward, Moving Forward." *Policy Studies Journal* 47 (2): 184–205.

Benamouzig, Daniel. 2005. *La santé au miroir de l'économie: Une histoire de l'économie de la santé en France.* Sociologies. Paris: Presses universitaires de France.

Benedetto, Giacomo, Simon Hix, and Nicola Mastrorocco. 2020. "The Rise and Fall of Social Democracy, 1918–2017." *American Political Science Review* 114 (3): 928–39.

Bénard, Pascal, Jean-Guy Hemono, Laurent Lester, and Yann Zennati. 2020. "Projet territorial de santé mentale du Morbihan – Feuille de route 2021–2025." Report prepared for l'Agence Régionale de Santé Bretagne.

Bennett, Andrew. 2010. "Process Tracing and Causal Inference." *Rethinking Social Inquiry: Diverse Tools, Shared Standards*, 2nd ed., edited by Henry E. Brady and David Collier, 207–20. Lanham: Rowman & Littlefield.

Bergeron, Henri. 1999. *L'État et la toxicomanie: Histoire d'une singularité française.* Paris: Presses universitaires de France.

Bertin, Giovanni, Ludovico Carrino, and Marta Pantalone. 2021. "Do Standard Classifications Still Represent European Welfare Typologies? Novel Evidence from Studies on Health and Social Care." *Social Science & Medicine* 281 (July): 114086.

Betz, Hans-Georg. 1994. *Radical Right-Wing Populism in Western Europe.* New York: St. Martin's Press.

Biarez, Sylvie. 2004. "Une politique publique: la santé mentale (1970–2002)." *Revue française d'administration publique* 111 (3): 517–31.

Birnbaum, Morton. 1960. "The Right to Treatment." *ABA Journal* 46 (May): 499–505.

Bishop, Tara F., Matthew J. Press, Salomeh Keyhani, and Harold Alan Pincus. 2014. "Acceptance of Insurance by Psychiatrists and the Implications for Access to Mental Health Care." *JAMA Psychiatry* 71 (2): 176–81.

BLS (Bureau of Labor Statistics). 2023. "CPI Inflation Calculator." www.bls.gov/data/inflation_calculator.htm.

Bode, Ingo. 2017. "Social Services in Post-Industrial Europe: An Incomplete Success Story and Its Tragic Moments." *Social Services Disrupted: Changes, Challenges and Policy Implications for Europe in Times of Austerity*, edited by Flavia Martinelli, Anneli Anttonen, and Margitta Matzke, 95–113. New Horizons in Social Policy. Cheltenham: Edward Elgar Publishing.

Boräng, Frida. 2018. *National Institutions–International Migration: Labour Markets, Welfare States and Immigration Policy.* London: Rowman & Littlefield.

Bouhallier, Gaspard. 2021. "'Pour que maman ne parte pas si loin' Familles de malades et personnel hospitalier face à la politique de rationalisation des dépenses en psychiatrie (1945–1948)." *Histoire, médecine et santé* 20: 155–78.

Brady, David, Evelyne Huber, and John D. Stephens. 2020. "Comparative Welfare States Dataset." University of North Carolina and WZB Berlin Social Science Center. https://huberandstephens.web.unc.edu/common-works/data/.

Brochmann, Grete. 2018. "Immigration Policies of the Scandinavian Countries." *The Routledge Handbook of Scandinavian Politics*, edited by Peter Nedergaard and Peter Wivel, 229–39. London: Routledge.

Brown, Phil. 1985. *The Transfer of Care: Psychiatric Deinstitutionalization and Its Aftermath*. London: Routledge & Kegan Paul.

Bueltzingsloewen, Isabelle von. 2007. *L'Hécatombe des fous: La famine dans les hôpitaux psychiatriques français sous l'Occupation*. Collection Historique. Paris: Aubier.

Busemeyer, Marius R., Aurélien Abrassart, and Roula Nezi. 2021. "Beyond Positive and Negative: New Perspectives on Feedback Effects in Public Opinion on the Welfare State." *British Journal of Political Science* 51 (1): 137–62.

Bussi, Margherita, Claire Dupuy, and Virginie Van Ingelgom. 2022. "Does Social Policy Change Impact on Politics? A Review of Policy Feedbacks on Citizens' Political Participation and Attitudes towards Politics." *Journal of European Social Policy* 32 (5): 607–18.

Cadeville, Olivier de. 2016. "Psychiatrie (RIM-P) – Bilan PMSI 2015." Activité des établissements: Les établissements bretons de santé. Agence Régionale de Santé Bretagne.

Cameron, David R. 1978. "The Expansion of the Public Economy: A Comparative Analysis." *American Political Science Review* 72 (4): 1243–61.

Campbell, Andrea Louise. 2003. *How Policies Make Citizens: Senior Political Activism and the American Welfare State*. Princeton Studies in American Politics. Princeton: Princeton University Press.

Capdevielle, Jacques, and René Moriaux. 1988. *Mai 68, L'entre-deux de la modernité. Histoire de trente ans*. Paris: Presses de la Fondation Nationale des Sciences Politiques.

Capoccia, Giovanni, and R. Daniel Kelemen. 2007. "The Study of Critical Junctures: Theory, Narrative, and Counterfactuals in Historical Institutionalism." *World Politics* 59 (3): 341–69.

Carpenter, Daniel P. 2001. *The Forging of Bureaucratic Autonomy: Reputations, Networks, and Policy Innovation in Executive Agencies, 1862–1928*. Princeton Studies in American Politics. Princeton: Princeton University Press.

Castell, Laura, and Céline Dennevault. 2017. "Qualité et accès aux soins: que pensent les français de leurs médecins." 1035. Études et Résultats. Direction de la recherche, des études, de l'évaluation et des statistiques.

Castles, Francis G. 2009. "What Welfare States Do: A Disaggregated Expenditure Approach." *Journal of Social Policy* 38 (1): 45–62.

Chapireau, François. 2021. "La désinstitutionnalisation psychiatrique: définitions, usages de la notion, et questions de méthode." *L'information psychiatrique* 97 (1): 39–43.

Chapireau, François. 2022. "Les patients aux pièges du financement départemental en psychiatrie: France 1838–1985." *L'information psychiatrique* 98 (6): 475–80.

Charlson, Fiona J., Alize J. Ferrari, Damian F. Santomauro et al., 2018. "'Global Epidemiology and Burden of Schizophrenia' Findings from the Global Burden of Disease Study 2016." *Schizophrenia Bulletin* 44 (6):1195–203.

Chevreul, Karine, Isabelle Durand-Zaleski, Stéphane Bahrami, Cristina Hernández-Quevedo, and Philipa Mladovsky. 2010. "France: Health System Review." *Health Systems in Transition* 12 (6): 1–291.

Chevreul, Karine, Karen Berg Brigham, Isabelle Durand-Zaleski, and Cristina Hernández-Quevedo. 2015. "France: Health System Review." *Health Systems in Transition* 17 (3): 1–218.

CHU Réseau. 2008. "Chapitre 2, 1958–1968, La création des centres hospitaliers et universitaires." *La grande histoire des CHU*, 39–65. www.chu-media.info/fileadmin/reseau-chu/user_upload/presentation_des_chus/chapitre_2.pdf.

Cingano, Federico. 2014. "Trends in Income Inequality and Its Impact on Economic Growth." OECD Social, Employment and Migration Working Papers 163. Vol. 163. OECD Social, Employment and Migration Working Papers.

Cléry-Melin, Philippe. 2002. "L'exercise de la psychiatrie libérale, hier et aujourd'hui." *Annales Médico-Psychologiques* 160: 794–98.

Coffin, Jean-Christophe. 2005. "'Misery' and 'Revolution:' The Organisation of French Psychiatry, 1900–1980." *Psychiatric Cultures Compared: Psychiatry and Mental Health Care in the Twentieth Century: Comparisons and Approaches*, edited by Marijke Gijswijt-Hofstra, Harry Oosterhuis, Joost Vijselaar, and Hugh Freeman, 225–47. Amsterdam: Amsterdam University Press.

Coldefy, Magali. 2007 "La prise en charge santé mentale: Recueil d'études statistiques." 07 096. Direction de la recherche, des études, de l'évaluation et des statistiques.

Coldefy, Magali. 2010. "De l'asile à la ville: une géographie de la prise en charge de la maladie mentale en France." Doctoral thesis, Université Panthéon-Sorbonne–Paris I.

Coldefy, Magali, Philippe Le Fur, Véronique Lucas-Gabrielli, and Julien Mousquès. 2009. "Cinquante ans de sectorisation psychiatrique en France: Des inégalités persistantes de moyens et d'organisation." Questions d'économie de la santé 145. Institut de recherche de documentation en économie de la santé.

Cole, Alistair. 2008. *Governing and Governance in France*. Cambridge: Cambridge University Press.

Collier, Ruth Berins, and Samuel Handlin, editors. 2009. *Reorganizing Popular Politics: Participation and the New Interest Regime in Latin America*. University Park: Pennsylvania State University Press.

Commissariat général du Plan. 1982. "Neuvième plan de développement économique, social et culturel (1984–1988)." La Documentation française.

Connery, Robert H. 1968. *The Politics of Mental Health: Organizing Community Mental Health in Metropolitan Areas*. New York: Columbia University Press.

Costabile, Antonio. 2009. *Legalità, manipolazione, democrazia : lineamenti del sistema politico meridionale*. Biblioteca di testi e studi; Studi politici 499. Rome: Carocci.

Cramer, Katherine J. 2016. *The Politics of Resentment: Rural Consciousness in Wisconsin and the Rise of Scott Walker*. Chicago Studies in American Politics. Chicago: University of Chicago Press.

Culhane, Dennis P. 2008. "The Cost of Homelessness: A Perspective from the United States." *European Journal of Homelessness* 2: 97–114.

Cunningham, Peter J. 2009. "Beyond Parity: Primary Care Physicians' Perspectives on Access to Mental Health Care." *Health Affairs* 28 (3): w490–501.

Cusack, Thomas R. 2004. "Public Finance Data for 20 OECD Countries." WZB (Berlin Social Research Center). www.wzb.eu/en/node/113/subpage/5662.

Dahlström, Carl. 2009. "The Bureaucratic Politics of Welfare-State Crisis: Sweden in the 1990s." *Governance* 22 (2): 217–38.

Daly, Mary, and Jane Lewis. 2000. "The Concept of Social Care and the Analysis of Contemporary Welfare States." *The British Journal of Sociology* 51 (2): 281–98.

Dear, Michael J., and Jennifer R Wolch. 1987. *Landscapes of Despair: From Deinstitutionalization to Homelessness*. Princeton: Princeton University Press.

Demay, Marie, and Jean Demay. 1982. "Une voie française pour une psychiatrie différente, document établi à la demande de M. Jack Ralite, Ministre de la santé."

Derrien, Marie, and Mathilde Rossigneux-Méheust. 2020. "L'État social à l'épreuve des personnes âgées atteintes de troubles mentaux: Une expérience de réadaptation pendant les années 1950." *20 & 21. Revue d'histoire* 145 (1): 19.

Deutsch, Albert. 1948. *The Shame of the States*. New York: Harcourt, Brace, and Company.

DGC (Directorate-General for Communication). 2014. "Special Eurobarometer 345: Mental Health." EU Open Data Portal. http://data.europa.eu/euodp/en/data/dataset/S898_73_2_EBS345.

Di Carlo, Donato. 2019. "The Political Economy of Public Sector Wage Setting in Europe." For the Max Planck Institute for the Study of Societies "Political Economy of Public Sector Wage Setting" Conference, Cologne.

Di Carlo, Donato. 2023. "Beyond Neo-Corporatism: State Employers and the Special-Interest Politics of Public Sector Wage-Setting." *Journal of European Public Policy* 30 (5): 967–94.

Diseth, Rigmor R. 2017. "Norsk psykiatri fra 'tinglovene' til i dag." *Michael* 14 (S20): 19–24.

Dixon, Keith. 2009. "Implementing Mental Health Parity: The Challenge for Health Plans." *Health Affairs* 28 (3): 663–65.

Donnelly, Michael. 1992. *The Politics of Mental Health in Italy*. London: Tavistock/Routledge.

Dowbiggin, Ian Robert. 1991. *Inheriting Madness: Professionalization and Psychiatric Knowledge in Nineteenth-Century France*. Medicine and Society. Berkeley: University of California Press.

DREES (Direction de la recherche, des études, de l'évaluation et des statistiques). 2016. "Les établissements de santé." Panoramas de la DREES Santé. Direction de la recherche, des études, de l'évaluation et des statistiques.

Druss, Benjamin G., Thomas Bornemann, Yvonne W. Fry-Johnson, Harriet G. McCombs, Robert M. Politzer, and George Rust. 2008. "Trends in Mental Health and Substance Abuse Services at the Nation's Community Health Centers: 1998–2003." *American Journal of Public Health* 98 (9 Suppl): S126–31.

Duggan, Maria, Ben Harris, Wai-Kwan Chislett, and Rosemary Calder. 2020. "Nowhere Else to Go: Why Australia's Health System Results in People Getting 'Stuck' in Emergency Departments." Mitchell Institute Commissioned Report for the Australasian College for Emergency Medicine. Victoria University.

Durkheim, Émile. 1897. *Le Suicide: Étude de Sociologie.* Paris: Félix Alcan.

Dutton, Paul V. 2008. *Differential Diagnoses.* Ithaca, NY: ILR Press.

ECB (European Central Bank). 2022. "Currency Converter." Statistical Data Warehouse. https://data.ecb.europa.eu/currency-converter.

Edwards-Grossi, Élodie. 2021. *Bad Brains: La psychiatrie et la lutte des Noirs américains pour la justice raciale, XXe-XXIe siècles.* Rennes: Presses universitaires de Rennes.

Emmenegger, Patrick, Silja Häusermann, Bruno Palier, and Rennes Seeleib-Kaiser, editors. 2012. *The Age of Dualization: The Changing Face of Inequality in Deindustrializing Societies.* International Policy Exchange Series. Oxford: Oxford University Press.

Erkulwater, Jennifer L. 2006. *Disability Rights and the American Social Safety Net.* Ithaca, NY: Cornell University Press.

Esping-Andersen, Gøsta. 1990. *The Three Worlds of Welfare Capitalism.* Princeton: Princeton University Press.

Esping-Andersen, Gøsta. 1999. *Social Foundations of Postindustrial Economies.* Oxford: Oxford University Press.

Estévez-Abe, Margarita. 2008. *Welfare and Capitalism in Postwar Japan: Party, Bureaucracy, and Business.* Cambridge Studies in Comparative Politics. Cambridge: Cambridge University Press.

Estévez-Abe, Margarita, Torben Iversen, and David Soskice. 2001. "Social Protection and the Formation of Skills: A Reinterpretation of the Welfare State." *Varieties of Capitalism,* edited by Peter A. Hall and David Soskice, 145–83. Oxford: Oxford University Press.

European Commission. 2010. "Second Biennial Report on Social Services of General Interest." Commission Staff Working Document SEC(2010) 1284 final. Publications Office of the European Union.

European Commission. 2014. "Special Supplement: Health and Social Services from an Employment and Economic Perspective." EU Employment and Social Situation Quarterly Review. Publications Office of the European Union.

Falleti, Tulia G., and Julia F. Lynch. 2009. "Context and Causal Mechanisms in Political Analysis." *Comparative Political Studies* 42 (9): 1143–66.

Faraggi, Pierre, and Benoît Dayot. 2016. "Marie Demay." *L'Information psychiatrique* 92 (3): 253–54.

Ferrera, Maurizio. 1996. "The 'Southern Model' of Welfare in Social Europe." *Journal of European Social Policy* 6 (1): 17–37.

Finger, Leslie K., and Carlos X. Lastra-Anadón. 2021. "Advocates for Hire: How Government Contracting Shapes Politics." *Governance* 35 (1): 187–208.

Fisher, William H., Jeffrey L. Geller, and John A. Pandiani. 2009. "The Changing Role of the State Psychiatric Hospital." *Health Affairs* 28 (3): 676–84.

FitzGerald, Chloë, and Samia Hurst. 2017. "Implicit Bias and Healthcare Professionals: A Systematic Review." *BMC Medical Ethics* 18 (19), 1–18.

Foley, Henry A. 1975. *Community Mental Health Legislation: The Formative Process.* Lexington, MA: Lexington Books.

Foot, John. 2015. *The Man Who Closed the Asylums: Franco Basaglia and the Revolution in Mental Health Care.* London: Verso.

Ford, Matt. 2015. "America's Largest Mental Hospital Is a Jail." *The Atlantic.* June 8, 2015.

Forman, Miloš. 1975. *One Flew Over the Cuckoo's Nest.* United Artists.

Foucault, Michel. 1961. *Folie et déraison: histoire de la folie à l'âge classique.* Paris: Plon.

Frank, Richard G., Chris Koyanagi, and Thomas G. McGuire. 1997. "The Politics and Economics of Mental Health 'Parity' Laws." *Health Affairs* 16 (4): 108–19.

Frank, Richard G., and Thomas G. McGuire. 2000. "Chapter 16 Economics and Mental Health." *Handbook of Health Economics*, vol. 1, edited by Anthony J. Cuyler and Joseph P. Newhouse, 893–954. Amsterdam: Elsevier.

Freeman, Richard B. 1988. "Contraction and Expansion: The Divergence of Private Sector and Public Sector Unionism in the United States." *Journal of Economic Perspectives* 2 (2): 63–88.

Frymer, Paul. 2005. "Racism Revised: Courts, Labor Law, and the Institutional Construction of Racial Animus." *American Political Science Review* 99 (3): 373–87.

Fuller Torrey, E., Doris A. Fuller, Jeffrey Geller, Carla Jacobs, and Kristina Ragosta. 2012. "No Room at the Inn: Trends and Consequences of Closing Psychiatric Hospitals, 2005–2010." Treatment Advocacy Center.

Gallois, Pierre, and Alain Taïb. 1981. "Rapport au ministre de la santé: De l'organisation du système de soins." La Documentation française.

Garfield, Rachel. 2011. "Mental Health Financing in the United States: A Primer." 8182. The Kaiser Commission on Medicaid and the Uninsured. The Henry J. Kaiser Family Foundation.

Garfield, Rachel L., Judith R. Lave, and Julie M. Donohue. 2010. "Health Reform and the Scope of Benefits for Mental Health and Substance Use Disorder Services." *Psychiatric Services* 61 (11): 1081–86.

Garrabé, Jean. 2005. "Théophile Kammerer (1917–2005)." *L'Évolution Psychiatrique* 70 (3): 663–64.

Garrett, Geoffrey, and Christopher Way. 1999. "Public Sector Unions, Corporatism, and Macroeconomic Performance." *Comparative Political Studies* 32 (4): 411–34.

Gay, Renaud. 2011. "Les réformes hospitalières au début des années 1980: une bifurcation du système hospitalier? Politisation de l'action publique et capacités réformatrices limitées." Quatrième congrès de l'association française de sociologie, Grenoble.

Gerring, John. 1999. "What Makes a Concept Good? A Criterial Framework for Understanding Concept Formation in the Social Sciences." *Polity* 31 (3): 357–93.

Gerring, John. 2014. *Case Study Research.* Cambridge: Cambridge University Press.

Giaimo, Susan. 2002. *Markets and Medicine: The Politics of Health Care Reform in Britain, Germany, and the United States.* Ann Arbor: University of Michigan Press.

Gilens, Martin. 1999. *Why Americans Hate Welfare: Race, Media, and the Politics of Antipoverty Policy.* Studies in Communication, Media, and Public Opinion. Chicago: University of Chicago Press.

Gillon, Steven M. 2000. *That's Not What We Meant to Do: Reform and Its Unintended Consequences in Twentieth-Century America.* New York: W. W. Norton.

Gingrich, Jane. 2011. *Making Markets in the Welfare State: The Politics of Varying Market Reforms.* Cambridge Studies in Comparative Politics. Cambridge: Cambridge University Press.

Gingrich, Jane, and Sara Watson. 2016. "Privatizing Participation? The Impact of Private Welfare Provision on Democratic Accountability." *Politics & Society* 44 (4): 573–613.

Gingrich, Jane, and Silja Häusermann. 2015. "The Decline of the Working-Class Vote, the Reconfiguration of the Welfare Support Coalition and Consequences for the Welfare State." *Journal of European Social Policy* 25 (1): 50–75.

Glenngärd, Anna H. 2020. "Sweden." International Health Care System Profiles: The Commonwealth Fund.

Goertz, Gary. 2020. *Social Science Concepts and Measurement.* Princeton: Princeton University Press.

Goffman, Erving. 1961. *Asylums: Essays on the Social Situation of Mental Patients and Other Inmates.* Garden City, NY: Anchor Books.

Golden, Miriam. 1993. "The Dynamics of Trade Unionism and National Economic Performance." *American Political Science Review* 87 (2): 439–54.

Goldstein, Jan Ellen. 1987. *Console and Classify: The French Psychiatric Profession in the Nineteenth Century.* Chicago: University of Chicago Press.

Goodwin, Simon. 1997. *Comparative Mental Health Policy: From Institutional to Community Care.* Thousand Oaks, CA: Sage Publications.

Gottschalk, Marie. 2006. *The Prison and the Gallows: The Politics of Mass Incarceration in America.* Cambridge Studies in Criminology. Cambridge: Cambridge University Press.

Gottschalk, Marie. 2012. "The Great Recession and the Great Confinement: The Economic Crisis and the Future of Penal Reform." *Contemporary Issues in Criminological Theory and Research – The Role of Social Institutions*, edited by Richard Rosenfeld, Kenna Quinet, and Crystal A. Garcia, 343–70. Belmont, CA: Wadsworth.

Gourevitch, Peter A., and James Shinn. 2007. *Political Power and Corporate Control: The New Global Politics of Corporate Governance.* Princeton: Princeton University Press.

Gourevitch, Peter Alexis. 1980. *Paris and the Provinces: The Politics of Local Government Reform in France.* London: George Allen & Unwin.

Grob, Gerald N. 1983. *Mental Illness and American Society, 1875–1940.* Princeton: Princeton University Press.

Grob, Gerald N. 1991. *From Asylum to Community: Mental Health Policy in Modern America.* Princeton: Princeton University Press.

Grob, Gerald N. 1994. *The Mad among Us: A History of the Care of America's Mentally Ill.* New York: Maxwell Macmillan International.

Grob, Gerald N. 2005. "Public Policy and Mental Illnesses: Jimmy Carter's Presidential Commission on Mental Health." *The Milbank Quarterly* 83 (3): 425–56.

Grob, Gerald N., and Howard H. Goldman. 2006. *The Dilemma of Federal Mental Health Policy: Radical Reform or Incremental Change?* New Brunswick, NJ: Rutgers University Press.

Gronfein, William. 1985. "Psychotropic Drugs and the Origins of Deinstitutionalization." *Social Problems* 32 (5): 437–54.

Guérin, Vincent. 2011. "'Ne plus être un monde à part': La transformation d'un hôpital psychiatrique: Sainte-Gemmes-Sur-Loire (1910–1977)." Doctoral thesis, Université d'Angers.

Gusmano, Michael K., Victor G. Rodwin, and Daniel Weisz. 2010. *Health Care in World Cities: New York, Paris, and London.* Baltimore: Johns Hopkins University Press.

Han, Hahrie. 2014. *How Organizations Develop Activists: Civic Associations and Leadership in the 21st Century.* Oxford University Press. https://doi.org/10.1093/acprof:oso/9780199336760.001.0001.

Hacker, Jacob S. 2002. *The Divided Welfare State: The Battle over Public and Private Social Benefits in the United States.* Cambridge: Cambridge University Press.

Hacker, Jacob S., Alexander Hertel-Fernandez, Paul Pierson, and Kathleen Ann Thelen, editors. 2021. *The American Political Economy: Politics, Markets, and Power.* Cambridge Studies in Comparative Politics. Cambridge: Cambridge University Press.

Hackett, Ursula. 2020. *America's Voucher Politics: How Elites Learned to Hide the State.* Cambridge: Cambridge University Press.

Hall, Peter A., and David W. Soskice, editors. 2001. *Varieties of Capitalism: The Institutional Foundations of Comparative Advantage.* Oxford: Oxford University Press.

Hall, William J., Mimi V. Chapman, Kent M. Lee, et al. 2015. "Implicit Racial/Ethnic Bias among Health Care Professionals and Its Influence on Health Care Outcomes: A Systematic Review." *American Journal of Public Health* 105 (12): e66–76.

Hansen, Martin Ejnar. 2018. "Cabinets and Ministerial Turnover in the Scandinavian Countries." *The Routledge Handbook of Scandinavian Politics,* edited by Peter Nedergaard and Peter Wivel, 92–102. London: Routledge.

Harcourt, Bernard E. 2011. "An Institutionalization Effect: The Impact of Mental Hospitalization and Imprisonment on Homicide in the United States, 1934–2001." *The Journal of Legal Studies* 40 (1): 39–83.

Häusermann, Silja. 2020. "Dualization and Electoral Realignment." *Political Science Research and Methods* 8 (2): 380–85.

Häusermann, Silja, and Hanna Schwander. 2012. "Varieties of Dualization? Labor Market Segmentation and Insider-Outsider Divides Across Regimes." *The Age of Dualization,* edited by Patrick Emmenegger, Silja Hausermann, Bruno Palier, and Martin Seeleib-Kaiser, 27–51. Oxford: Oxford University Press.

Henckes, Nicolas. 2007. "Le nouveau monde de la psychiatrie française: Les psychiatres, l'État et la réforme des hôpitaux psychiatriques de l'après-guerre aux années 1970." Doctoral, Paris: École des hautes études en sciences sociales.

Henckes, Nicolas. 2009. "Narratives of Change and Reform Processes: Global and Local Transactions in French Psychiatric Hospital Reform after the Second World War." *Social Science & Medicine* 68 (3): 511–18.

Henckes, Nicolas. 2011a. "La politique du handicap psychique. Familles, psychiatres et État face à la chronicité des maladies mentales des années 1960 aux années 1970." Rapport de recherche Drees-MiRe, Convention de Recherche 2547. Paris: CERMES3.

Henckes, Nicolas. 2011b. "Reforming Psychiatric Institutions in the Mid-Twentieth Century: A Framework for Analysis." *History of Psychiatry* 22 (2): 164–81.

Hermann, Christoph, and Jörg Flecker. 2015. *Privatization of Public Services: Impacts for Employment, Working Conditions, and Service Quality in Europe.* London: Routledge.

Hochschild, Arlie Russell. 2018. *Strangers in Their Own Land: Anger and Mourning on the American Right.* New York: The New Press.

Honkapohja, Seppo. 2009. *The 1990's Financial Crises in Nordic Countries.* Bank of Finland Research Discussion Paper No. 5. Helsinki: Bank of Finland.

Houston, Megan. 2023. "Medicaid's Institution for Mental Disease (IMD) Exclusion." Congressional Research Service.

Howard, Christopher. 1997. *The Hidden Welfare State: Tax Expenditures and Social Policy in the United States.* Princeton Studies in American Politics. Princeton: Princeton University Press.

Huber, Evelyne, and John D. Stephens. 2000. "Partisan Governance, Women's Employment, and the Social Democratic Service State." *American Sociological Review* 65 (3): 323–42.

Huber, Evelyne, and John D. Stephens. 2001. *Development and Crisis of the Welfare State: Parties and Policies in Global Markets.* Chicago: University of Chicago Press.

Immergut, Ellen M. 1992. *Health Politics: Interests and Institutions in Western Europe.* Cambridge Studies in Comparative Politics. Cambridge: Cambridge University Press.

INSEE (Institut nationale de la statistique et des études économiques). 2023. "Convertisseur franc-euro." www.insee.fr/fr/information/2417794.

Iversen, Torben, and Anne Wren. 1998. "Equality, Employment, and Budgetary Restraint: The Trilemma of the Service Economy." *World Politics* 50 (4): 507–46.

Jacobs, Alan M., and R. Kent Weaver. 2015. "When Policies Undo Themselves: Self-Undermining Feedback as a Source of Policy Change." *Governance* 28 (4): 441–57.

Jacobs, Lawrence R. 1993. *The Health of Nations: Public Opinion and the Making of American and British Health Policy.* Ithaca, NY: Cornell University Press.

Jaeger, Marcel. 1989. *La psychiatrie en France.* Paris: Syros-Alternatives.

James, Doris J., and Lauren E. Glaze. 2006. "Mental Health Problems of Prison and Jail Inmates." Special Report NCJ 213600. US Department of Justice, Office of Justice Programs, Bureau of Justice Statistics.

Jensen, Carsten. 2008. "Worlds of Welfare Services and Transfers." *Journal of European Social Policy* 18 (2): 151–62.

Jensen, Carsten. 2011. "Determinants of Welfare Service Provision after the Golden Age: Determinants of Welfare Service Provision." *International Journal of Social Welfare* 20 (2): 125–34.

Jensen, Gail A., Kathryn Rost, Russell P. D. Burton, and Maria Bulycheva. 1998. "Mental Health Insurance in the 1990s: Are Employers Offering Less to More?" *Health Affairs* 17 (3): 201–8.

Joel, Billy. 1982. "Allentown." *The Nylon Curtain*, CBS.

Johnson, Sheri L., Erik Wibbels, and Richard Wilkinson. 2015. "Economic Inequality Is Related to Cross-National Prevalence of Psychotic Symptoms." *Social Psychiatry and Psychiatric Epidemiology* 50 (12): 1799–807.

Joint Commission on Mental Illness and Health. 1961. *Action for Mental Health*. New York: Basic Books.

Jones, Kathleen. 1983. "Services for the Mentally Ill: The Death of Concept." *Approaches to Welfare*, edited by Philip Bean and Stewart MacPherson, 218–34. Routledge Library Editions. Welfare and the State. London: Routledge.

Jones, Kathleen. 1993. *Asylums and After: A Revised History of the Mental Health Services: From the Early 18th Century to the 1990s*. London: Athlone Press.

Karavokyros, Dimitri. 2010. "Le role du syndicat des médecins des hôpitaux psychiatriques dans la mise en place du secteur." *Érès* 1 (25): 97–104.

Katz, Michael B. 1996. *In the Shadow of the Poorhouse: A Social History of Welfare in America*. 10th anniversary ed. New York: Basic Books.

Katz Olson, Laura. 2010. *The Politics of Medicaid*. New York: Columbia University Press.

Kautto, Mikko. 2002. "Investing in Services in West European Welfare States." *Journal of European Social Policy* 12 (1): 53–65.

Kersbergen, Kees van. 1995. *Social Capitalism: A Study of Christian Democracy and the Welfare State*. London: Routledge.

Kesey, Ken. 1962. *One Flew Over the Cuckoo's Nest*. New York: Viking Press.

King, Desmond S. 1987. *The New Right: Politics, Markets and Citizenship*. London: Macmillan.

King, Desmond S. 1995. *Actively Seeking Work? The Politics of Unemployment and Welfare Policy in the United States and Great Britain*. Chicago: University of Chicago Press.

Kirk, Stuart A., and Herb Kutchins. 1992. *The Selling of DSM: The Rhetoric of Science in Psychiatry*. Social Problems and Social Issues. New York: Aldine de Gruyter.

Kjellberg, Anders, and Kristine Nergaard. 2022. "Union Density in Norway and Sweden: Stability versus Decline." *Nordic Journal of Working Life Studies* 12 (S8): 51–72.

Kohn, Robert, Ali Ahsan Ali, Victor Puac-Polanco, Chantal Figueroa, Victor López-Soto, Kristen Morgan, Sandra Saldivia, and Benjamín Vicente. 2018. "Mental Health in the Americas: An Overview of the Treatment Gap." *Revista Panamericana de Salud Pública* 42: e165.

Korpi, Walter. 1983. *The Democratic Class Struggle*. London; Boston: Routledge & Kegan Paul.

Kramer, Morton. 1977. "Psychiatric Services and the Changing Institutional Scene, 1950–1985." US Department of Health, Education, and Welfare, Public Health Service, Alcohol, Drug Abuse, and Mental Health Administration.

Kritsotaki, Despo, Vicky Long, and Matthew Smith, editors. 2016. *Deinstitutionalisation and after: Post-War Psychiatry in the Western World*. Mental Health in Historical Perspective. Cham: Palgrave Macmillan.

Laegrid, Per. 2018. "Nordic Administrative Traditions." *The Routledge Handbook of Scandinavian Politics*, edited by Peter Nedergaard and Peter Wivel, 229–39. London: Routledge.

Laing, Ronald David. 1960. *The Divided Self.* London: Tavistock Publications.

Laird, Jennifer. 2017. "Public Sector Employment Inequality in the United States and the Great Recession." *Demography* 54 (1): 391–411.

Lara-Millán, Armando. 2021. *Redistributing the Poor: Jails, Hospitals, and the Crisis of Law and Fiscal Austerity.* Oxford: Oxford University Press.

Lauzier, J., and D. Lafage. 1958. "Statistiques médicales des hôpitaux psychiatriques et des dispensaires d'hygiène mentale." *Bulletin de l'Institut national d'hygiène* 15 (3): 437–57.

Leguay, Denis. 2002. "Le système de soins psychiatriques français: réalités et perspectives." Mulhouse: Congrès de psychiatrie et de neurologie de langue française.

Lerman, Paul. 1982. *Deinstitutionalization and the Welfare State.* New Brunswick, NJ: Rutgers University Press.

Levi, Margaret, David Olson, Jon Agnone, and Devin Kelly. 2009. "Union Democracy Reexamined." *Politics & Society* 37 (2): 203–28.

Levy, Jonah D. 1999. *Tocqueville's Revenge: State, Society, and Economy in Contemporary France.* Cambridge, MA: Harvard University Press.

Lieberman, Robert C. 1998. *Shifting the Color Line: Race and the American Welfare State.* Cambridge, MA: Harvard University Press.

Lieberman, Robert C. 2003. "Race and the Limits of Solidarity: American Welfare State Development in Comparative Perspective." *Race and the Politics of Welfare Reform,* edited by Sanford Schram, Joe Soss, and Richard C. Fording, 23–46. Ann Arbor: University of Michigan Press.

Lindert, Peter H. 2004. *Growing Public: Social Spending and Economic Growth since the Eighteenth Century.* Cambridge: Cambridge University Press.

Lindqvist, Rafael. 2012. *Funktionshindrade i välfärdssamhället.* 3rd ed. Malmö: Gleerups.

Lipsky, Michael. 1980. *Street-Level Bureaucracy: Dilemmas of the Individual in Public Services.* Publications of Russell Sage Foundation. New York: Russell Sage Foundation.

Litvak, Anatole. 1948. *The Snake Pit.* 20th Century Fox.

Longin, Y. 1999. "Petite histoire des hôpitaux psychiatriques français." *L'Évolution Psychiatrique* 64 (3): 611–25.

Lopez, Alain, and Gaëlle Turan-Pelletier. 2017. "Organisation et fonctionnement du dispositif de soins psychiatriques, 60 ans après la circulaire du 15 mars 1960." 2017-064R. Inspection générale des affaires sociales.

Lynch, Julia. 2020. *Regimes of Inequality: The Political Economy of Health and Wealth.* Cambridge: Cambridge University Press.

Lyons, Amelia H. 2013. *The Civilizing Mission in the Metropole: Algerian Families and the French Welfare State during Decolonization.* Redwood City, CA: Stanford University Press.

Mahoney, James, and Gary Goertz. 2004. "The Possibility Principle: Choosing Negative Cases in Comparative Research." *American Political Science Review* 98 (4): 653–69.

Mahoney, James, and Kathleen Thelen, eds. 2009. "A Theory of Gradual Institutional Change." *Explaining Institutional Change,* 1–37. Cambridge: Cambridge University Press.

Mahoney, James, and P. Larkin Terrie. 2008. "Comparative-Historical Analysis in Contemporary Political Science." *Oxford Handbook of Political Methodology*, edited by Henry Brady, Janet M. Box-Steffenmeier, and David Collier, 737–55. Oxford: Oxford University Press.

Maioni, Antonia. 1998. *Parting at the Crossroads*. Princeton Studies in American Politics. Princeton: Princeton University Press.

Malm, Ulf, Lars Jacobsson, and Nils O. Larsson. 2002. "Psychiatry in Sweden: Values, System, and Evidence for a Reform in Progress." *International Journal of Mental Health* 31 (4): 50–65.

Manderscheid, Ron. 2009. "Effects of Mental Health Parity." *Health Affairs* 28 (4): 1228.

Mares, Isabela. 2003. *The Politics of Social Risk: Business and Welfare State Development*. Cambridge Studies in Comparative Politics. Cambridge: Cambridge University Press.

Markström, Urban. 2003. "Den Svenska Psykiatrireformen: Bland Brukare, Eldsjälar Och Byråkratar." Doctoral, Umeå.

Markström, Urban. 2019. "Stöd till Personer Med Psykisk Funktionsnedsättning." *Socialvetenskaplig Tidskrift* 26 (3–4): 323–40.

Markström, Urban. 2020. "Det samhällsbaserade arbetet efter institutionerna." *Att leva med psykisk funktionsnedsättning: livssituation och effektiva vård- och stödinsatser*, edited by David Brunt, Ulrika Bejerholm, Urban Markström, and Lars Hansson, 63–78. Lund: Studentlitteratur AB.

Markström, Urban, Mikael Sandlund, and Rafael Lindqvist. 2003. "Who Is Responsible for Supporting 'Long-Term Mentally Ill' Persons?: Reforming Mental Health Practices in Sweden." *Canadian Journal of Community Mental Health* 23 (2): 51–63.

Markström, Urban, and Rafael Lindqvist. 2015. "Establishment of Community Mental Health Systems in a Postdeinstitutional Era: A Study of Organizational Structures and Service Provision in Sweden." *Journal of Social Work in Disability & Rehabilitation* 14 (2): 124–44.

Martin, Cathie Jo, and Duane Swank. 2012. *The Political Construction of Business Interests: Coordination, Growth, and Equality*. Cambridge Studies in Comparative Politics. Cambridge: Cambridge University Press.

Martin, Jean-Pierre. 2004. "La politique à l'épreuve de la psychiatrie." *Revue internationale de psychosociologie* X (22): 51–63.

Martinelli, Flavia. 2017. "Social Services, Welfare States and Places: An Overview." *Social Services Disrupted: Changes, Challenges and Policy Implications for Europe in Times of Austerity*, edited by Flavia Martinelli, Anneli Anttonen, and Margitta Matzke, 11–48. New Horizons in Social Policy. Cheltenham: Edward Elgar Publishing.

Martinelli, Flavia, Anneli Anttonen, and Margitta Matzke, editors. 2017. *Social Services Disrupted: Changes, Challenges and Policy Implications for Europe in Times of Austerity*. New Horizons in Social Policy. Cheltenham: Edward Elgar Publishing.

Maycraft Kall, Wendy Katherine. 2010. "The Governance Gap: Central-Local Steering and Mental Health Reform in Britain and Sweden." Doctoral, Uppsala: Uppsala.

Mayes, Rick, and Allan V. Horwitz. 2005. "DSM-III and the Revolution in the Classification of Mental Illness." *Journal of the History of the Behavioral Sciences* 41 (3): 249–67.

McAdam, Doug, Sidney Tarrow, and Charles Tilly. 2001. *Dynamics of Contention.* Cambridge Studies in Contentious Politics. Cambridge: Cambridge University Press.

McGovern, Constance M. 1985. *Masters of Madness: Social Origins of the American Psychiatric Profession.* Hanover, NH: Published for University of Vermont by University Press of New England.

Mechanic, David, and David A. Rochefort. 1990. "Deinstitutionalization: An Appraisal of Reform." *Annual Review of Sociology* 16 (1): 301–27.

Meslé, France, and Jacques Vallin. 1981. "La population des établissements psychiatriques: évolution de la morbidité ou changement de stratégie médicale?" *Population* 36 (6): 1035–68.

Mettler, Suzanne. 1998. *Dividing Citizens: Gender and Federalism in New Deal Public Policy.* Ithaca, NY: Cornell University Press.

Mettler, Suzanne. 2005. *Soldiers to Citizens: The G.I. Bill and the Making of the Greatest Generation.* Oxford: Oxford University Press.

Mettler, Suzanne. 2011. *The Submerged State: How Invisible Government Policies Undermine American Democracy.* Chicago Studies in American Politics. Chicago: University of Chicago Press.

Mettler, Suzanne, and Joe Soss. 2004. "The Consequences of Public Policy for Democratic Citizenship: Bridging Policy Studies and Mass Politics." *Perspectives on Politics* 2 (1): 55–73.

Metzl, Jonathan. 2009. *The Protest Psychosis: How Schizophrenia Became a Black Disease.* Boston: Beacon Press.

Michener, Jamila. 2018. *Fragmented Democracy: Medicaid, Federalism, and Unequal Politics.* Cambridge: Cambridge University Press.

Mill, John Stuart. 1874. *A System of Logic, Ratiocinative and Inductive.* 8th ed. New York: Harper & Brothers.

Mitchell, Alison. 2016. "Medicaid Disproportionate Share Hospital Payments." 7–5700; R42865. Congressional Research Service.

Moe, Terry M. 2006. "Political Control and the Power of the Agent." *The Journal of Law, Economics, and Organization* 22 (1): 1–29.

Moe, Terry M. 2011. *Special Interest: Teachers Unions and America's Public Schools.* Washington, DC: Brookings Institution Press.

Molina, Oscar. 2014. "Self-Regulation and the State in Industrial Relations in Southern Europe: Back to the Future?" *European Journal of Industrial Relations* 20 (1): 21–36.

Moran, Michael. 2000. "Understanding the Welfare State: The Case of Health Care." *British Journal of Politics and Industrial Relations* 2 (2): 135–60.

Morgan, Kimberly J. 2005. "The 'Production' of Child Care: How Labor Markets Shape Social Policy and Vice-Versa." *Social Politics: International Studies in Gender, State & Society* 12 (2): 243–63.

Morgan, Kimberly J. 2006. *Working Mothers and the Welfare State: Religion and the Politics of Work-Family Policies in Western Europe and the United States.* Stanford: Stanford University Press.

Morgan, Kimberly J., and Andrea Louise Campbell. 2005. "Federalism and the Politics of Old-Age Care in Germany and the United States." *Comparative Political Studies* 38 (8): 887–914.

Morgan, Kimberly J., and Andrea Louise Campbell. 2011. *The Delegated Welfare State: Medicare, Markets, and the Governance of Social Policy.* Oxford Studies in Postwar American Political Development. New York: Oxford University Press.

Mori, Anna. 2020. *Employment Relations in Outsourced Public Services Working Between Market and State.* Cham: Palgrave.

Mosley, Layna, editor. 2013. *Interview Research in Political Science.* Ithaca, NY: Cornell University Press.

Mossé, Philippe, and Robert Tchobanian. 1999. "France: The Restructuring of Employment Relations in the Public Services." *Public Service Employment Relations in Europe: Transformation, Modernization or Inertia?* edited by Stephen Bach, Lorenzo Bordogna, Giuseppe Della Rocca, and David Winchester, 130–63. London: Routledge.

Mossialos, Elias, Ana Djordjevic, and Robin Osborn. 2017. "International Profiles of Health Care Systems." The Commonwealth Fund.

Mossman, Douglas. 1997. "Deinstitutionalization, Homelessness, and the Myth of Psychiatric Abandonment: A Structural Anthropology Perspective." *Social Science & Medicine* 44 (1): 71–83.

Mudde, Cas. 2000. *The Ideology of the Extreme Right.* Manchester: Manchester University Press.

Mudge, Stephanie L. 2018. *Leftism Reinvented: Western Parties from Socialism to Neoliberalism.* Cambridge, MA: Harvard University Press.

Murard, Lion, and François Fourquet, editors. 1975. *Histoire de la psychiatrie de secteur ou le secteur impossible?* Paris: Recherches.

Naczyk, Marek. 2013. "Agents of Privatization? Business Groups and the Rise of Pension Funds in Continental Europe." *Socio-Economic Review* 11 (3): 441–69.

NASMHPD (National Association of State Mental Health Program Directors). 2018. "About Us." 2018. www.nasmhpd.org/content/about-us.

Nijhuis, Dennie Oude. 2013. *Labor Divided in the Postwar European Welfare State: The Netherlands and the United Kingdom.* Cambridge: Cambridge University Press.

NIMH (National Institute of Mental Health). 1977. "Private Psychiatric Hospitals, 1974–1975." 18. A. Mental Health Facility Reports. US Department of Health, Education, and Welfare.

NIMH (National Institute of Mental Health). n.d. "Mental Illness." Accessed September 26, 2021. www.nimh.nih.gov/health/statistics/mental-illness.

Niskanen, William A. 1971. *Bureaucracy and Representative Government.* Chicago: Aldine, Atherton.

NOMESCO-NOSOSCO (Nordic Medico-Statistical Committee and Nordic Social Statistical Committee). 2022. "Health care user charges." Nordic Health and Welfare Statistics. https://nhwstat.org/health/organization-health-services/health-care-user-charges.

Norges Bank. 2023a. "Exchange Rates." www.norges-bank.no/en/topics/Statistics/exchange_rates/?tab=currency&id=USD.

Norges Bank. 2023b. "Price Calculator." www.norges-bank.no/en/topics/Statistics/Price-calculator-/.

Obinger, Herbert, and Peter Starke. 2015. "Welfare State Transformation: Convergence and the Rise of the Supply-Side Model." *The Oxford Handbook of Transformations of the State*, edited by Stephan Leibfried, Evelyne Huber, Matthew Lange, Jonah D. Levy, and John D. Stephens, 465–81. Oxford: Oxford University Press.

Obinger, Herbert, Stephan Leibfried, and Francis Geoffrey Castles, editors. 2005. *Federalism and the Welfare State: New World and European Experiences*. Cambridge: Cambridge University Press.

OEA (Office of European Analysis). 1983. "Mitterrand's Economic Management: Have the Lessons Been Learned? An Intelligence Assessment." EUR 83-10277. US Directorate of Intelligence.

OECD (Organisation for Economic Co-operation and Development). 2014. "The Netherlands Has an Innovative Mental Health System, but High Bed Numbers Remain a Concern." www.oecd.org/els/health-systems/MMHC-Country-Press-Note-Netherlands.pdf.

OECD (Organisation for Economic Co-operation and Development). 2021. *Government at a Glance 2021*. Paris: OECD Publishing.

OECD (Organisation for Economic Co-operation and Development). 2023. "Purchasing Power Parities." https://data.oecd.org/conversion/purchasing-power-parities-ppp.htm.

Oesch, Daniel. 2006. *Redrawing the Class Map*. Basingstoke: Palgrave Macmillan.

Oesch, Daniel, and Line Rennwald. 2018. "Electoral Competition in Europe's New Tripolar Political Space: Class Voting for the Left, Centre-Right and Radical Right." *European Journal of Political Research* 57 (4): 783–807.

Ohlsson, Anna. 2008. "Myt Och Manipulation: Radikal Psykiatrikritik i Svensk Offentlig Idédebatt 1968–1973." Doctoral, University of Stockholm.

Olfson, Mark, and Steven C. Marcus. 2010. "National Trends in Outpatient Psychotherapy." *American Journal of Psychiatry* 167 (12): 1456–63.

Oliver, Rebecca J. 2011. "Powerful Remnants? The Politics of Egalitarian Bargaining Institutions in Italy and Sweden." *Socio-Economic Review* 9 (3): 533–66.

Oorschot, Wim van, Femke Roosma, Bart Meuleman, and Tim Reeskens, editors. 2017. *The Social Legitimacy of Targeted Welfare: Attitudes to Welfare Deservingness*. Globalization and Welfare. Cheltenham: Edward Elgar Publishing.

Pan, Deanna. 2013. "Timeline: Deinstitutionalization and Its Consequences." *Mother Jones*. April 29, 2013.

Parsons, Anne E. 2018. *From Asylum to Prison: Deinstitutionalization and the Rise of Mass Incarceration after 1945*. Justice, Power, and Politics. Chapel Hill: The University of North Carolina Press.

Parsons, Talcott. 1951. *The Social System*. New York: The Free Press.

Patashnik, Eric M. 2008. *Reforms at Risk: What Happens after Major Policy Changes Are Enacted*. Princeton Studies in American Politics. Princeton: Princeton University Press.

PCMH (President's Commission on Mental Health). 1978. "Report to the President." US Government Printing Office.

Penrose, Lionel S. 1939. "Mental Disease and Crime: Outline of a Comparative Study of European Statistics." *British Journal of Medical Psychology* 18 (1): 1–15.

Perera, Isabel M. 2019. "Is Psychiatry Different? An Economic Perspective." *The Lancet Psychiatry* 6 (4): 282–83.

Perera, Isabel M. 2020a. "The Relationship between Hospital and Community Psychiatry: Complements, Not Substitutes?" *Psychiatric Services* 71 (January): 964–66.

Perera, Isabel M. 2020b. "Two Dogmas of Mental Health Policy." *Health Affairs Blog* (blog). March 2, 2020.

Perera, Isabel M. 2020c. "Complements, Not Substitutes? Reply to Smith and Saxena Commentaries." *Psychiatric Services* 71 (12): 1322.

Perera, Isabel M. 2022. "Interest Group Governance and Policy Agendas." *Governance* 35 (3): 869–86.

Perera, Isabel M., and Trevor Brown. In press. "Why States Do or Do Not Privatize: Cross-Class Coalitions in the Public Sector." *World Politics*.

Petersson, Olof. 2016. "Rational Politics: Commissions of Inquiry and the Referral System in Sweden." *The Oxford Handbook of Swedish Politics*, edited by Jon Pierre, 650–62. Oxford: Oxford University Press.

Piel, Eric, and Jean-Luc Roelandt. 2001. "De la psychiatrie vers la santé mentale." Rapport de Mission. Ministère de l'emploi et de la solidarité, Ministère délégué à la santé.

Pierson, Paul. 1994. *Dismantling the Welfare State? Reagan, Thatcher, and the Politics of Retrenchment*. Cambridge Studies in Comparative Politics. Cambridge: Cambridge University Press.

Pierson, Paul. 1996. "The New Politics of the Welfare State." *World Politics* 48 (2): 143–79.

Pierson, Paul. 2000a. "Not Just What, but *When*: Timing and Sequence in Political Processes." *Studies in American Political Development* 14 (1): 72–92.

Pierson, Paul. 2000b. "Increasing Returns, Path Dependence, and the Study of Politics." *American Political Science Review* 94 (2): 251–67.

Pierson, Paul, editor. 2001. *The New Politics of the Welfare State*. Oxford: Oxford University Press.

Pierson, Paul. 2004. *Politics in Time: History, Institutions, and Social Analysis*. Princeton: Princeton University Press.

Pit-ten Cate, Ineke M., and Sabine Cook. 2019. "Teachers' Implicit Attitudes toward Students from Different Social Groups: A Meta-Analysis." *Frontiers in Psychology* 10, Article 2832.

Piven, Frances Fox, and Richard A. Cloward. 1979. *Poor People's Movements: Why They Succeed, How They Fail*. New York: Vintage Books.

Ploeg, Frederick van der. 2007. "Sustainable Social Spending and Stagnant Public Services: Baumol's Cost Disease Revisited." *FinanzArchiv* 63 (4): 519.

Pontusson, Jonas. 2005. *Inequality and Prosperity: Social Europe vs. Liberal America*. Cornell Studies in Political Economy. Ithaca, NY: Cornell University Press.

Pontusson, Jonas, and Lucio Baccaro. 2020. "Comparative Political Economy and Varieties of Macroeconomics." *Oxford Research Encyclopedia of Politics*, edited by William R. Thompson, 1–27. Oxford: Oxford University Press. https://doi-org.eui.idm.oclc.org/10.1093/acrefore/9780190228637.013.161.

Pouvourville, Gérard de. 1986. "Hospital Reforms in France under a Socialist Government." *The Milbank Quarterly* 64 (3): 392–413.

Prasad, Monica. 2006. *The Politics of Free Markets: The Rise of Neoliberal Economic Policies in Britain, France, Germany, and the United States*. Chicago: University of Chicago Press.

Prince, Martin, editor. 2018. "Forum: Measuring and Improving the Quality of Mental Health Care." *World Psychiatry* 17 (1): 30–48.

Quadagno, Jill S. 1994. *The Color of Welfare: How Racism Undermined the War on Poverty*. Oxford: Oxford University Press.

Rathgeb, Philip. 2021. "Makers against Takers: The Socio-Economic Ideology and Policy of the Austrian Freedom Party." *West European Politics* 44 (3): 635–60.

Rehm, Philipp. 2020. "The Future of Welfare State Politics." *Political Science Research and Methods* 8 (2): 386–90.

Reibling, Nadine. 2010. "Healthcare Systems in Europe: Towards an Incorporation of Patient Access." *Journal of European Social Policy* 20 (1): 5–18.

Reynaud, Michel, Alain Lopez, and André-Julien Coudert. 1994. *Evaluation et organisation des soins en psychiatrie*. Paris: Frison-Roche.

Rice, Thomas, Pauline Rosenau, Lynn Y. Unruh, and Andrew J. Barnes. 2013. "United States of America: Health System Review." *Health Systems in Transition* 15 (3): 1–431.

Riksbank. 2022. "Cross Rates." www.riksbank.se/en-gb/statistics/search-interest--exchange-rates/cross-rates/.

Robcis, Camille. 2021. *Disalienation: Politics, Philosophy, and Radical Psychiatry in Postwar France*. Chicago Studies in Practices of Meaning. Chicago: University of Chicago Press.

Rocco, Philip, and Chloe Thurston. 2014. "From Metaphors to Measures: Observable Indicators of Gradual Institutional Change." *Journal of Public Policy* 34 (1): 35–62.

Rochefort, David A. 1993. *From Poorhouses to Homelessness: Policy Analysis and Mental Health Care*. Westport, CT: Auburn House.

Rodwin, Victor. 1982. "Management without Objectives: The French Health Policy Gamble." *The Public/Private Mix for Health*, edited by Gordon McLachlan and Alan Maynard, 289–325. London: Nuffield Provincial Hospitals Trust.

Roelcke, Volker, Paul Weindling, and Louise Westwood, editors. 2010. *International Relations in Psychiatry: Britain, Germany, and the United States to World War II*. Rochester Studies in Medical History, v. 16. Rochester: University of Rochester Press.

Rogers, Katren. 2022. "Party Ideology and Care Services: The Decline of Institutional Care since 1950." Presented at the Council of European Studies Annual Meeting. Lisbon.

Romøren, Tor Inge. 2018. "Spesialisthelsetjenesten: sykehus og psykisk hel-severn." *Den norske velferdsstaten*, edited by Aksel Hatland, Stein Kuhnle, and Tor Inge Romøren, 149–77. Oslo: Gyldendal.

Rothman, David J. 1971. *The Discovery of the Asylum: Social Order and Disorder in the New Republic*. Boston: Little, Brown.

Rothman, David J. 1980. *Conscience and Convenience: The Asylum and Its Alternatives in Progressive America*. Boston: Little, Brown.

Rueda, David. 2007. *Social Democracy Inside Out: Partisanship and Labor Market Policy in Industrialized Democracies*. Oxford: Oxford University Press.

Rueda, David. 2014. "Dualization, Crisis and the Welfare State." *Socio-Economic Review* 12 (2): 381–407.

Safon, Marie-Odile. 2017. "Les réformes hospitalières en France: aspects historiques et réglementaires, synthèse documentaire." Institut de recherche de documentation en économie de la santé.

Sainsbury, Diane. 2012. *Welfare States and Immigrant Rights: The Politics of Inclusion and Exclusion*. Oxford: Oxford University Press.

Salamon, Lester M. 1995. *Partners in Public Service: Government-Nonprofit Relations in the Modern Welfare State*. Baltimore: Johns Hopkins University Press.

SAMHSA (Substance Abuse and Mental Health Services Administration). 1992. "Mental Health, United States, 1992." SMA-92-1942. US Department of Health and Human Services, Substance Abuse and Mental Health Services Administration.

SAMHSA (Substance Abuse and Mental Health Services Administration). 2011. "Funding and Characteristics of State Mental Health Agencies, 2009." SMA-11-4655. Substance Abuse and Mental Health Services Administration.

SAMHSA (Substance Abuse and Mental Health Services Administration). 2012. "Mental Health, United States, 2010." SMA-12-4681. US Department of Health and Human Services, Substance Abuse and Mental Health Services Administration.

SAMHSA (Substance Abuse and Mental Health Services Administration). 2014. "Highlights of the National Mental Health Services Survey, 2010." Substance Abuse and Mental Health Services Administration, Center for Behavioral Health Statistics and Quality.

SCB (Statistikmyndigheten). 2023. "CPI, Fixed Index Numbers." www.scb .se/en/finding-statistics/statistics-by-subject-area/prices-and-consumption/ consumer-price-index/consumer-price-index-cpi/pong/tables-and-graphs/ consumer-price-index-cpi/cpi-fixed-index-numbers-1980100/.

Scheff, Thomas J. 1966. *Being Mentally Ill: A Sociological Theory*. Chicago: Aldine.

Scheff, Thomas J. 2014. "A Note on the Origins of Deinstitutionalization." *Deviant Behavior* 35 (6): 475–76.

Schmidt, Vivien. 2003. "French Capitalism Transformed, Yet Still a Third Variety of Capitalism." *Economy and Society* 32 (4): 526–54.

Schmitter, Philippe, and Wolfgang Streeck. 1999. "The Organization of Business Interests: Studying the Associative Action of Business in Advanced Industrial Societies." MpifG Discussion Paper 99/1. Max Planck Institute for the Study of Societies.

Schofield, William. 1964. *Psychotherapy: The Purchase of Friendship*. Englewood Cliffs, NJ: Prentice-Hall.

Schuknecht, Ludger. 2020. *Public Spending and the Role of the State: History, Performance, Risk and Remedies*. Cambridge: Cambridge University Press.

Scull, Andrew. 1984. *Decarceration: Community Treatment and the Deviant: A Radical View*. 2nd ed. New Brunswick, NJ: Rutgers University Press.

Seeleib-Kaiser, Martin, Adam Saunders, and Marek Naczyk. 2012. "Shifting the Public-Private Mix." *The Age of Dualization*, edited by Patrick Emmenegger, Silja Hausermann, Bruno Palier, and Martin Seeleib-Kaiser, 151–75. Oxford: Oxford University Press.

Sharfstein, Steven S., and Harry W. Clark. 1978. "Economics and the Chronic Mental Patient." *Schizophrenia Bulletin* 4 (3): 399–414.

Sheingate, Adam D. 2001. *The Rise of the Agricultural Welfare State: Institutions and Interest Group Power in the United States, France, and Japan*. Princeton Studies in American Politics. Princeton: Princeton University Press.

Shepard, Todd. 2008. *The Invention of Decolonization: The Algerian War and the Remaking of France*. Ithaca, NY: Cornell University Press.

Silfverhielm, Helena, and Claes Göran Stefansson. 2006. "Sweden." *International Psychiatry: Bulletin of the Board of International Affairs of the Royal College of Psychiatrists* 3 (1): 9–12.

Silfverhielm, Helena, and Edna Kamis-Gould. 2000. "The Swedish Mental Health System." *International Journal of Law and Psychiatry* 23 (3–4): 293–307.

Singh, Prerna, and Matthias Vom Hau. 2016. "Ethnicity in Time: Politics, History, and the Relationship between Ethnic Diversity and Public Goods Provision." *Comparative Political Studies* 49 (10): 1303–40.

Siwek-Pouydesseau, Jeanne. 1989. *Les syndicats des fonctionnaires depuis 1948*. Paris: Presses universitaires de France.

Skocpol, Theda. 1992. *Protecting Soldiers and Mothers: The Political Origins of Social Policy in the United States*. Cambridge, MA: Belknap Press of Harvard University Press.

Skowronek, Stephen. 1982. *Building a New American State: The Expansion of National Administrative Capacities, 1877–1920*. Cambridge: Cambridge University Press.

Slater, Dan, and Daniel Ziblatt. 2013. "The Enduring Indispensability of the Controlled Comparison." *Comparative Political Studies* 46 (10): 1301–27.

Slater, Dan, and Erica Simmons. 2010. "Informative Regress: Critical Antecedents in Comparative Politics." *Comparative Political Studies* 43 (7): 886–917.

SNAC (Social Networks and Archival Context). n.d. "Santiestevan, Henry." University of Virginia Library and National Archives and Records Administration. Accessed January 11, 2024. http://n2t.net/ark:/99166/w6ot2288.

Soifer, Hillel. 2020. "Shadow Cases in Comparative Research." *Qualitative and Multi-Method Research* 18 (2): 9–18.

Soss, Joe. 1999. "Lessons of Welfare: Policy Design, Political Learning, and Political Action." *American Political Science Review* 93 (2): 363–80.

Sotiropoulos, Dimitri A. 2004. "Southern European Public Bureaucracies in Comparative Perspective." *West European Politics* 27 (3): 405–22.

Sperre Saunes, Ingrid. 2020. "Norway." *International Health Care System Profiles*. New York: The Commonwealth Fund. www.commonwealthfund.org/international-health-policy-center/countries/norway.

SPF (Svenska Psykiatriska Föreningen). 1992. "Svensk psykiatri på väg mot 2000-talet." White Paper.

Steadman, Henry J., John Monahan, Barbara Duffee, Eliot Hartstone, and Pamela Clark Robbins. 1984. "The Impact of State Mental Hospital Deinstitutionalization on United States Prison Populations, 1968–1978." *The Journal of Criminal Law and Criminology* 75 (2): 474–90.

Stephens, John D. 1979. *The Transition from Capitalism to Socialism*. New Studies in Sociology. London: Macmillan.

Stokes, Susan Carol. 2013. *Brokers, Voters, and Clientelism: The Puzzle of Distributive Politics*. Cambridge Studies in Comparative Politics. Cambridge: Cambridge University Press.

Stone, Deborah A. 1984. *The Disabled State*. Philadelphia: Temple University Press.

Stoy, Volquart. 2014. "Worlds of Welfare Services: From Discovery to Exploration." *Social Policy & Administration* 48 (3): 343–60.

Streeck, Wolfgang. 2013. "The Politics of Public Debt: Neoliberalism, Capitalist Development, and the Restructuring of the State." MPIfG Discussion Paper 13/7. Cologne: Max Planck Institute for the Study of Societies.

Streeck, Wolfgang. 2017. *Buying Time: The Delayed Crisis of Democratic Capitalism*. Translated by Patrick Camiller and David Fernbach. 2nd ed. London New York: Verso.

Swenson, Peter A. 2002. *Capitalists against Markets*. Oxford: Oxford University Press.

Swenson, Peter A. 2018. "Misrepresented Interests: Business, Medicare, and the Making of the American Health Care State." *Studies in American Political Development* 32 (1): 1–23.

Swenson, Peter A. 2021. *Disorder: A History of Reform, Reaction, and Money in American Medicine*. New Haven: Yale University Press.

Szasz, Thomas S. 1961. *The Myth of Mental Illness: Foundations of a Theory of Personal Conduct*. New York: Harper & Row.

Szasz, Thomas S. 1970. *The Manufacture of Madness, a Comparative Study of the Inquisition and the Mental Health Movement*. New York: Harper & Row.

Tarrow, Sidney. 2010. "The Strategy of Paired Comparison: Toward a Theory of Practice." *Comparative Political Studies* 43 (2): 230–59.

Tarrow, Sidney G. 1994. *Power in Movement: Social Movements, Collective Action, and Politics*. Cambridge Studies in Comparative Politics. Cambridge: Cambridge University Press.

Tartour, Tonya. 2021. "L'administration du désordre. Gouverner l'hôpital psychiatrique depuis les années 1980." Doctoral thesis, Sciences Po Paris.

Thachil, Tariq. 2014. *Elite Parties, Poor Voters: How Social Services Win Votes in India*. Cambridge: Cambridge University Press.

The Lancet [Editorial Staff]. 2016. "The Health Crisis of Mental Health Stigma." *The Lancet* 387 (10023): 1027.

Thelen, Kathleen A. 2004. *How Institutions Evolve: The Political Economy of Skills in Germany, Britain, the United States, and Japan*. Cambridge Studies in Comparative Politics. Cambridge: Cambridge University Press.

Thornicroft, Graham, and Michele Tansella. 2013. "The Balanced Care Model: The Case for Both Hospital- and Community-Based Mental Healthcare." *British Journal of Psychiatry* 202 (2): 246–48.

Thurston, Chloe N. 2018. *At the Boundaries of Homeownership: Credit, Discrimination, and the American State.* Cambridge: Cambridge University Press.

Tilly, Charles. 1986. *The Contentious French.* Cambridge, MA: Harvard University Press.

Toloudis, Nicholas. 2012. *Teaching Marianne and Uncle Sam: Public Education, State Centralization, and Teacher Unionism in France and the United States.* Politics, History, and Social Change. Philadelphia: Temple University Press.

Torrey, E. Fuller. 1988. *Nowhere to Go: The Tragic Odyssey of the Homeless Mentally Ill.* New York: Harper & Row.

Tuohy, Carolyn H. 2018. *Remaking Policy: Scale, Pace, and Political Strategy in Health Care Reform.* Toronto: University of Toronto Press.

USP (Union syndicale de la psychiatrie, formerly Syndicat de la psychiatrie). 2021. "L'USP, un demi siècle d'histoire." Union syndicale de la psychiatrie (website). www.uspsy.fr/?p=26654.

Vail, Mark I. 2010. *Recasting Welfare Capitalism: Economic Adjustment in Contemporary France and Germany.* Philadelphia: Temple University Press.

Van Evera, Stephen. 1997. *Guide to Methods for Students of Political Science.* Ithaca, NY: Cornell University Press.

Vincent, Catherine. 2016. "France: The Crisis Speeds Up Public Service Reform and Adjustment." *Public Service Management and Employee Relations in Europe: Emerging from the Crisis,* edited by Stephen Bach and Lorenzo Bordogna, 112–25. New York: Routledge.

Walker, Alexis N. 2020. *Divided Unions: The Wagner Act, Federalism, and Organized Labor.* American Governance: Politics, Policy, and Public Law. Philadelphia: University of Pennsylvania Press.

Ward, Mary Jane. 1946. *The Snake Pit.* New York: Random House.

Weaver, Kent. 2010. "Paths and Forks or Chutes and Ladders?: Negative Feedbacks and Policy Regime Change." *Journal of Public Policy* 30 (2): 137–62.

Weir, Margaret, Ann Shola Orloff, and Theda Skocpol, eds. 1988. *The Politics of Social Policy in the United States.* Studies from the Project on the Federal Social Role. Princeton: Princeton University Press.

Weir, Margaret, and Theda Skocpol. 1985. "State Structures and the Possibilities for 'Keynesian' Responses to the Great Depression in Sweden, Britain, and the United States." *Bringing the State Back In,* edited by Peter B. Evans, Dietrich Rueschemeyer, and Theda Skocpol, 107–64. Cambridge: Cambridge University Press.

Wendt, Claus, and Clare Bambra. 2020. "From Ideal Types to Health Care System Typologies: Dimensions, Labels, and Country Classifications." *Ideal Types in Comparative Social Policy,* edited by Christian Aspalter, 169–86. New York: Routledge.

WHO (World Health Organization). 1978. "The Future of Mental Hospitals: Report on a Working Group; Mannheim; 2–5 November 1976." Copenhagen: Regional Office for Europe.

WHO (World Health Organization). 2011. "Mental Health Atlas 2011." www .who.int/mental_health/publications/mental_health_atlas_2011/en/.

WHO (World Health Organization). 2014a. "Innovation in Deinstitutionalization: A WHO Expert Survey." World Health Organization and the Calouste Gulbenkian Foundation.

WHO (World Health Organization). 2014b. *Social Determinants of Mental Health*. https://iris.who.int/handle/10665/112828.

WHO (World Health Organization). 2022. "Schizophrenia." www.who.int/news-room/fact-sheets/detail/schizophrenia.

Wilfahrt, Martha. 2022. *Precolonial Legacies in Postcolonial Politics: Representation and Redistribution in Decentralized West Africa*. Cambridge Studies in Comparative Politics. Cambridge: Cambridge University Press.

Willison, Charley E., and Amanda I. Mauri. 2021. "Urban Homeless Policy in OECD Nations." *Oxford Research Encyclopedia of Global Public Health*, edited by David V. McQueen. Oxford: Oxford University Press.

Wilsford, David. 1991. *Doctors and the State: The Politics of Health Care in France and the United States*. Durham: Duke University Press.

Wilson, George, Vincent J. Roscigno, and Matt Huffman. 2015. "Racial Income Inequality and Public Sector Privatization." *Social Problems* 62 (2): 163–85.

Witkin, Michael J., Joanne Atay, and Ronald W. Manderscheid. 1996. "Trends in State and County Mental Hospitals in the US from 1970 to 1992." *Psychiatric Services* 47 (10): 1079–81.

Wren, Anne, editor. 2013. *The Political Economy of the Service Transition*. Oxford: Oxford University Press.

Zur, Julia, MaryBeth Musumeci, and Rachel Garfield. 2017. "Medicaid's Role in Financing Behavioral Health Services for Low-Income Individuals." Kaiser Family Foundation.

Zwan, Natascha van der. 2014. "Making Sense of Financialization." *Socio-Economic Review* 12 (1): 99–129.

Index

Cambridge Studies in Comparative Politics

OTHER BOOKS IN THE SERIES (*continued from page ii*)

Sven Steinmo, *The Evolution of Modern States: Sweden, Japan, and the United States*

Sven Steinmo, Kathleen Thelen, and Frank Longstreth, eds., *Structuring Politics: Historical Institutionalism in Comparative Analysis*

Susan C. Stokes, *Mandates and Democracy: Neoliberalism by Surprise in Latin America*

Susan C. Stokes, ed., *Public Support for Market Reforms in New Democracies*

Susan C. Stokes, Thad Dunning, Marcelo Nazareno, and Valeria Brusco, *Brokers, Voters, and Clientelism: The Puzzle of Distributive Politics*

Milan W. Svolik, *The Politics of Authoritarian Rule*

Duane Swank, *Global Capital, Political Institutions, and Policy Change in Developed Welfare States*

David Szakonyi *Politics for Profit: Business, Elections, and Policymaking in Russia*

Sidney Tarrow, *Power in Movement: Social Movements and Contentious Politics*

Sidney Tarrow, *Power in Movement: Social Movements and Contentious Politics, Revised and Updated Third Edition*

Sidney Tarrow, *Power in Movement: Social Movements and Contentious Politics, Revised and Updated Fourth Edition*

Tariq Thachil, *Elite Parties, Poor Voters: How Social Services Win Votes in India*

Kathleen Thelen, *How Institutions Evolve: The Political Economy of Skills in Germany, Britain, the United States, and Japan*

Kathleen Thelen, *Varieties of Liberalization and the New Politics of Social Solidarity*

Charles Tilly, *Trust and Rule*

Daniel Treisman, *The Architecture of Government: Rethinking Political Decentralization*

Guillermo Trejo, *Popular Movements in Autocracies: Religion, Repression, and Indigenous Collective Action in Mexico*

Guillermo Trejo and Sandra Ley, *Votes, Drugs, and Violence: The Political Logic of Criminal Wars in Mexico*

Rory Truex, *Making Autocracy Work: Representation and Responsiveness in Modern China*

Lily L. Tsai, *Accountability without Democracy: How Solidary Groups Provide Public Goods in Rural China*

Lily L. Tsai, *When People Want Punishment: Retributive Justice and the Puzzle of Authoritarian Popularity*

Joshua Tucker, *Regional Economic Voting: Russia, Poland, Hungary, Slovakia and the Czech Republic, 1990–1999*

Ashutosh Varshney, *Democracy, Development, and the Countryside*

Yuhua Wang, *Tying the Autocrat's Hand: The Rise of the Rule of Law in China*

Jeremy M. Weinstein, *Inside Rebellion: The Politics of Insurgent Violence*

Andreas Wiedemann, *Indebted Societies: Credit and Welfare in Rich Democracies*

Martha Wilfahrt, *Precolonial Legacies in Postcolonial Politics: Representation and Redistribution in Decentralized West Africa*

Stephen I. Wilkinson, *Votes and Violence: Electoral Competition and Ethnic Riots in India*

Andreas Wimmer, *Waves of War: Nationalism, State Formation, and Ethnic Exclusion in the Modern World*

For EU product safety concerns, contact us at Calle de José Abascal, 56–1°,
28003 Madrid, Spain or eugpsr@cambridge.org.

www.ingramcontent.com/pod-product-compliance
Ingram Content Group UK Ltd.
Pitfield, Milton Keynes, MK11 3LW, UK
UKHW022040061225
465726UK00013B/983